Caring:
The Compassionate Healer

Caring:
The Compassionate Healer

Delores A. Gaut
Madeleine M. Leininger
Editors

CARING
iA PASSAGE
TO THE
"O' HEART

Center for Human Caring

National League for Nursing Press • New York
Pub. No. 15-2401

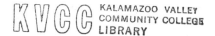

APR 1 3 1992

Copyright © 1991
National League for Nursing Press
350 Hudson Street, New York, NY 10014

ISBN 0-88737-518-9

This book was set in Goudy by Publications Development Company. The editor and designer was Allan Graubard. Clarkwood Corporation was the printer and binder. The cover was designed by Lillian Welsh.

Printed in the United States of America

Contents

Contributors

Ruth Ann Belknap, MSN, RN, Doctoral Student, Wayne State University, Detroit, Michigan, and Instructor, School of Nursing, Medical College of Ohio, Toledo, Ohio.

Carolyn L. Brown, PhD, RN, Assistant Professor, School of Nursing, Florida Atlantic University, Boca Raton, Florida.

Nassif J. Cannon, MD, Staff Physician, Cooper Green Hospital, Birmingham, Alabama.

Marylin J. Dodd, PhD, RN, FAAN, Professor, University of California, San Francisco, California.

Mary-Therese Dombeck, PhD, RNCS, Assistant Professor, School of Nursing, University of Rochester, Rochester, New York.

Sara T. Fry, PhD, RN, FAAN, Associate Professor, School of Nursing, University of Maryland, Baltimore, Maryland.

Delores A. Gaut, PhD, RN, Visiting Professor, University of Portland, Portland, Oregon, and President of the International Association for Human Caring.

Doris S. Greiner, MSN, RN, CS, Associate Professor, University of Alabama School of Nursing, Birmingham, Alabama.

Sigridur Halldorsdottir, MSN, RN, Assistant Professor, University of Iceland, Reykjavik, Iceland.

Linda Joseph, RN, BSN, Master's Candidate, School of Nursing, Florida Atlantic University, Boca Raton, Florida.

Patricia J. Larson, DNS, RN, Assistant Professor, University of California, San Francisco, California.

Carol Picard, MSCS, RN, Assistant Professor, Litchburg State College, Litchburg, Massachusetts.

Marilyn A. Ray, PhD, RN, Eminent Scholar, The Christine E. Lynn Endowed Chair in Nursing, Florida Atlantic University, Boca Raton, Florida.

Sister M. Simone Roach, PhD, RN, Mission Education Coordinator, St. Johns Hospital, Lowell, Massachusetts.

Gwen Sherwood, PhD, RN, Assistant Dean for Educational Outreach, School of Nursing, University of Texas Health Science Center, Houston, Texas.

Kathleen L. Valentine, PhD, RN, Director, Nursing Education and Research, Mary Imogene Bassett Hospital, Cooperstown, New York.

Bonnie Wesorick, MSN, RN, President CPM Resource Center, Grand Rapids, Michigan, and Project Director for Clinical Practice Model, Butterworth Hospital, Grand Rapids, Michigan.

Preface

Burgeoning technology in today's health care marketplace, cost conscious bureaucracies, and a prolonged nursing shortage have created a vacuum in caring relationships. There is a striving among health caregivers for a connectedness with others, for a culture of caring in organizational structures, for the high touch with the high technology. There is indeed a call to consciousness, a call to get in touch, a call to caring for the compassionate healer.

The day-to-day walk of the nurse, whatever the setting, is one of human contact, of meeting basic human needs. Believing that caring is the moral ideal of nursing, the University of Texas Health Science Center at Houston School of Nursing entered into a co-sponsorship with the International Association for Human Caring for the Twelfth Annual Human Caring Conference. That conference, held in Houston, Texas, in April 1990, addressed the theme, "Caring: The Compassionate Healer, A Call to Consciousness." This book is a direct result of that conference for the purpose of aiding growth and development of the compassionate healer through the reporting of systematic study of caring as the central and essential construct in professional nursing. Both the attendance at the conference and the evaluations of the participants validate the importance of this focus of study.

Health care professionals are taught to respect human life, protect human dignity, and maintain a person-centered approach in practice. Yet, increasingly, a focus on the bottom line, lack of support from administration, and time constraints have resulted in a conflict of values. Awareness of the moral duty to care inherent in any caregiving profession contrasted with the lack of

recognition for a practice grounded in caring constructs leave nurses disillu-
sioned, demoralized, and dissatisfied with the profession. The present reward
structure and incentives lead one to conclude that the emphasis is on cost-
cutting, time-efficient, nursing practice.

As we approach the last decade of the twentieth century and anticipate the
challenges of the future, it is clear that caring is becoming the legitimate and
accepted core of nursing. Therefore, a systematic study of caring from the
perspectives of theory, practice, and research is imperative. It is evident that
systematic study of caring is leading to identification of the operational
parameters of caring and advancement of theoretical models of caring. Data
analyses are providing descriptions of attributes patients desire and recognize
as inherent in a caring practice. As a highly visible and marketable commodity,
nursing must seize the opportunity to demonstrate the benefits of a caring
practice. The value of caring is being empirically linked with recovery as well
as with patient satisfaction and quality of care. This book adds to that expanding body of knowledge.

The compassionate healer is a caring presence not only at the traditional
bedside but also in the workplace and in society. It becomes a lifestyle of
living out one's sense of purpose, of total living, of respect for human
dignity in all situations. Humanness of the caregiver means a need for
continual renewal of strength to share with others; we won't all be 100
percent all the time. However, through systematic study and development
of the concept, we can know and promote strategies for living within a
holistic framework. Helping each other and those entrusted to our care
forms the core of the compassionate healer and is the essence of professional nursing. Growth and development of the compassionate healer is a
vital factor in retention of personnel. Assisting colleagues in living out their
life's purpose and professional identity helps to ensure their continuation of
the day-by-day challenge of health care delivery. That is the ultimate purpose of this book.

Caring is intentional human action. The compassionate healer, through
existential presencing, experiences awareness of needs, completes intentional,
skillful actions to meet those needs, and offers continual availability to the
other for assessment and interventions. We can, by promoting systematic
study of caring and by communicating and applying the learned results, enable
and empower the compassionate healer to implement a culture of caring
throughout our health care delivery system.

It is our challenge to reaffirm and sustain a model of caring in our practice,
both among colleagues and patients. The encouragement of self-expression as
exemplified in the establishment of annual caring conferences is instrumental

in helping the compassionate healer to fulfill that mission and goal, thus discovering the full potential of caring, the central construct of the nursing profession.

Gwen Sherwood, PhD, RN
Assistant Dean for Educational Outreach
The University of Texas
Health Science Center at Houston
School of Nursing

Patricia L. Starck, DSN, RN
Professor and Dean
The University of Texas
Health Science Center at Houston
School of Nursing

Foreword

It is most encouraging to see nurses becoming more involved in the full discovery and use of research findings focused on human care phenomena. Human care as the essence of nursing and the distinct, central, and coherent dimension of nursing has, at last, become our major focus. The importance of this development cannot be overlooked. In helping nurses to discover and value the significance of care, it has also helped in establishing and maintaining care as central to the discipline and profession of nursing.

Again, it is most encouraging to see nurses discover, value, and practice humanistic and scientific care to promote the healing and well being of those they serve. Of course, there are nurses who have been long committed to humanistic care because they experienced or saw the therapeutic values of such care in practice. These nurses have realized that care is the "heart and soul" of nursing, and that sundry other tasks must not deter them from providing quality based care. But there are other nurses who are discovering, perhaps for the first time in their career, the meaning and significance of care. These nurses are being taught and mentored to practice and value humanistic and scientific dimensions of care. Such different awarenesses reflect changing eras in nursing as traditional beliefs and commitments become reactivated, or as entirely new discoveries and insights about care became known to nurses. These trends also reflect differences among nurses in professional views and practices related to human caring.

During the past decade, it has also been fascinating to observe that lay people and especially business leaders have been attracted to the use of the terms *care* or *caring* to promote their work or products. Care has entered the public sector and has become of common linguistic usage. However, care has yet to enter fully into the world of politicians, economists, educators, and transnational entrepreneurs.

It has been my long standing hope that care would not only be institution-alized as a cultural norm in nursing and in all health professional endeavors, but also as a global care agenda. A global care agenda that goes beyond national or particular countries could revolutionize the world as a truly caring one. It could be the underlying basis for Bush's "New World Order" to promote peace and well being among all peoples and cultures. A global care agenda seems right for this post-Middle East War era. It is an agenda that must be transculturally based to accommodate the diversities and commonalities of human care expressions and values. For me, this cultural movement and goal to make care a professional nursing and worldwide commitment has been a lifetime endeavor. For it was in the late 1940s that I saw and valued the importance of care to healing, well being, and recovery from illness states; I envisioned that human care needed to be a transcultural and transpersonal focus. Today, human caring is becoming a reality in teaching, research, and practice. It is most encouraging to see young and eager nurses discover the full nature, meanings, and uses of care in a variety of nursing contexts. The cultural care movement is leading to a groundswell of new and different interests about care ranging from physical and technical care to transcultural and transcendental dimensions of care. This diversity of interest in studying care has lead to many different ways to understand and practice professional nursing. It has become the new and intense focus of nursing research and to new ways to teach and practice humanistic care.

A good share of the collective group impetus for the cultural care move-ment began with my initiation of the National Research Care Conferences with a cadre of interested care scholars in 1978. These care scholars became the major force to nurture and promote human care in nursing. In 1988, this organization was renamed the International Association of Human Caring (IAHC) because of a worldwide focus on human care with nurses and other scholars in advancing and discovering care knowledge, teaching, and practices. As a consequence, this international organization is stimulating many nurses and multidisciplinary colleagues to share their ideas, theories, research find-ings, and clinical experiences with one another as a community of care schol-ars. The in-depth perspectives of the many dimensions of human care are providing new cultural awarenesses about the power and relevance of care to professional nurses and to different disciplines. Most assuredly, it is creating a new ethos or driving force to make care the lasting and meaningful essence of nursing.

It is encouraging to see these care scholars and leaders to be helpful reflec-tors and constructive critics of those speakers, writers, and users of care rhetoric in order to advance care knowledge and its uses in diverse ways. Some of our care scholars continue to question and deplore ambiguous public media statements, such as, "If caring were enough, anyone could be a nurse." For this statement and others, we want care to be made clear to the public and to prevent any negative images, misunderstandings, or misinterpretations about human care and its importance. Most of all, care scholars do not want care practices and meanings to reflect devalued feminists activities.

This book focuses on the construct of compassion as healing. It is a major contribution to the evolving body of human care knowledge. The several contributors to this book reflect their creative discoveries and fresh viewpoints about compassion and its relationship to healing. Compassion as healing was a major care theme of the 1990 Houston, Texas, Conference. It was a most timely theme for the participants in that they seemed ready to focus on compassion as another area about care that had received limited attention. Although compassion had long been the unspoken expectation and norm of professional nursing practice since the days of Florence Nightingale, still the diversity of meanings and expressions had not been studied. This book, therefore, examines different dimensions of compassion and its relationship to caring, healing, and nursing. It is a publication that will help nurses think anew about compassion to understand and to view healing in new perspectives. For, indeed, students of human care continue to raise questions such as: "Is compassion a universal phenomenon among all cultures and caregivers?" "Is compassion a 'given' that one is born with?" "Is compassion something that can be learned?" What accounts for compassionate caregivers who so effectively promote healing with individuals and groups? Do "noncompassionate" or "cold-hearted" nurses or practitioners belong in the nursing profession? Can therapeutic or beneficial healing occur without expressions of compassion? How is compassion communicated to others in music, art, and literature? Can compassion be researched and taught? These questions and many others reflect how much there is yet to be learned about compassion as a caring modality. Undoubtedly, care scholars and students will continue to unravel the many mysteries about compassion in order to know and practice compassionate care. Comparative or transcultural meanings and expressions of compassion are essential for the full understanding of compassion, and especially as a global care agenda interest.

Most assuredly, the recent war in the Persian Gulf has made us think about human behavior. The brutal acts and atrocities committed against other human beings contrast sharply in our minds with those compassionate nurses, doctors, and paramedics who preserved life and displayed valiant expressions of compassion toward enemies as well as friends in the battle field. The experience of compassionate and noncompassionate behavior in war became alive and meaningful through home televisions, newspapers, and other public media. The moral and ethical aspects of compassion and what constitutes human compassion as justices, injustices, and "just war" remain alive in our minds. Nonetheless, it was difficult for most people to understand compassionate and noncompassionate acts during the Persian Gulf War. This war brought into awareness new meanings and ideas about compassion that will continue to influence our thinking and research interest on this phenomenon. Unquestionably, nursing will continue to hold a deep interest in compassion as central to promote healing and well being. Nurses will need, however, to forge ahead to understand transcultural aspects of human compassion with individuals, families, and institutions. Studies related to compassion with the dying, loss of body parts or functions, mental conflicts, political and economic oppression, daily life stresses, world hunger, and cultural conditions all need far more investigation. Most importantly, students of compassion will need to learn more directly from consumers how they know and experience compassion in the various vicissitudes of living.

One might proclaim that what the world needs most today is human compassion. However, our knowledge is imprecise and our practices are largely unknown of what constitutes compassion. Compassion is, however, more than an attitude. It is a knowledge domain that needs to be fully understood and with role models to demonstrate compassion, and to be taught, communicated, and evaluated. This book explores a few of these many queries and ideas about human compassion.

This book can be viewed as a means to help the reader gain theoretical insights and new perspectives about compassion by care research and scholars and to stimulate new thinkers and doers in the field. It is another major contribution to establish care as the essence and central unifying dimension of nursing. It is a means to encourage others to value care and to help establish a global care agenda as a worldwide cultural movement to influence all aspects of human caring. This publication should be helpful in establishing further the epistemic, philosophical, cultural, and clinical practices related to human care with the goal to advance or improve nursing care education, research, and practice about the science and humanistic aspects of care.

Madeleine Leininger, PhD, DS, RN, CTN, LHD, FAAN,
Co-Editor, Leader in Human Care Research and Teaching,
Founder of Transcultural Nursing Field

Introduction

Nurse scholars from around the world gathered together in Houston, Texas, with a common purpose and a common voice—to share knowledge and experiences in an attempt to reaffirm the dimension of compassion in caring. In 1989, as the board of directors discussed future visions for the caring research conferences, the growing numbers of vulnerable human beings in the world today demanded our attention.

The call went out for research and theoretical papers that would explicate the dimension of compassion in caring, examine the role of the nurse as the compassionate healer, and describe the impact of caring expressions in the lives of patients. The first five chapters address the dimension of compassion in caring.

Sister M. Simone Roach (Chapter 2) in the introductory keynote address, "The Call to Consciousness: Compassion in Today's Health World," set the tone of the conference. She called on participants to ponder, reflect on, and explore the meaning of human care. She challenged all nurses to professionalize the human capacity to care through compassion, competence, confidence, conscience, and commitment to caring as a human mode of being.

In Chapter 3, "The Contexts of Caring: Conscience and Consciousness," Mary-Therese Dombeck, building on Roach's previous work, focused on "conscience" as an essential mode of expression in the contexts of caring encounters. A theoretical framework is provided for describing and analyzing levels of moral awareness in such encounters.

Sigridur Halldorsdottir (Chapter 4), in "Five Basic Modes of Being with Another," suggested that modes of being with another in our world involve both caring and noncaring dimensions. By analyzing two of her own studies on clients' perceptions of caring and noncaring encounters, the author suggests five basic modes of being with another: life-giving, life-sustaining, life-neutral, life-restraining, and life-destroying.

Linda Joseph (Chapter 5), in "The Energetics of Conscious Caring for the Compassionate Healer," focused on the nurse as compassionate healer. She proposed that as nurses consciously integrate an understanding of the energy dynamics involved in caring for another, the barriers to and hazards of caring presences minimize. The energetics of knowing and caring presented in the works of Carper, Rogers, Parse, and Watson provided the theoretical context for this paper.

The next five papers describe the impact of caring expressions in the lives of patients. Patricia J. Larson and Marylin J. Dodd studied the "Cancer Family's Caring Experience" (Chapter 6). The study demonstrated that caring occurs and can be described in terms of contextual issues and patterns related to the cancer experience of a family member. It also demonstrated that for some cancer patients there are families who cannot provide caring.

Gwen Sherwood (Chapter 7), in an attempt to enhance understanding of professional nurse caring from the patient's perspective, conducted an inductive qualitative study in a group of postoperative patients. Her paper, "Expressions of Nurse's Caring: The Role of the Compassionate Healer," suggested that patients value caring as an essential part of nursing and that nursing is both doing and being in a dual aspect of skillful competence with a person-centered interactional approach.

Carol Picard (Chapter 8) in a unique approach, "Caring and the Story," focused on the use of stories as an avenue for more fully understanding the meaning of suffering and illness in a patient's life. The paper assessed what is understood about the patient's story and how stories from literature and film can help patients in expressing their suffering.

Kathleen L. Valentine (Chapter 9) presented a study, "Nurse–Patient Caring," that explored the relationships between patient experiences of caring and health outcomes and the degree to which it occurred in patient–nurse encounters. The results challenge conventional beliefs which many nurses may hold about caring and caring actions.

Utilizing a case history, Doris S. Greiner and Nassif J. Cannon (Chapter 10) shared their personal and continual reawakening to the consciousness and antecedent dynamics of caring. In "I Sent Myself A Card Today," the authors suggested a process of interior movements such as knowing, silence, stillness, and attentively receiving the story of persons being in the world. Such movements to assure sincere caring are necessary to become compassionate healers.

The next two papers discuss issues related to creating an environment that supports professional caring. Carolyn L. Brown (Chapter 11), in "Caring in Nursing Administration," suggested that nurse administrators, by virtue of their position, often hold the key to power for nurses in health care delivery systems. From her research, Brown concluded that nurse administrators also hold the key to the way caring, as the essence of nursing, is lived in health care systems. The nurse administrator who is committed to caring also empowers his or her nursing staff, thus promoting health and growth for individuals and organizations.

Bonnie Wesorick (Chapter 12) presented a clinical practice model that interfaces the dreams of caring theory with the clinical realities of nursing practice. In her paper, "Creating an Environment that Supports Professional Caring Service," she discussed approaches taken to create such environments by ten different hospitals located in eight different states. The author reviewed contemporary components of the practice model and suggested that the success of such a model is related to the support of the core beliefs of professional caring and shared governance.

The last three papers focus on the theoretical and scientific aspects of nursing as caring. Sara T. Fry (Chapter 13), in her keynote address, "A Theory of Caring: Pitfalls and Promises," briefly traced the development of the National Caring Research Conferences and the resultant scholarship on the phenomenon of caring and suggested future moves for theory development. From a review of some traditional models of care and caring, she explored hypothetical models of caring for the practice of nursing and described problems yet to be overcome in the development of theory adequate to address the multidimensional phenomena of caring.

Ruth Ann Belknap, in "Care: A Significant Paradigm Shift and Focus in Nursing for the Future" (Chapter 14), explored the intellectual movement in nursing wherein the concept of human care is becoming recognized as a central focus and major component in nursing's scheme for understanding and explaining reality. She suggested that as care emerges as the focus of the discipline, it would become evident that now, as throughout history, the healing power of the nurse is the result of her ability to provide compassionate human care.

Last, Marilyn A. Ray, in "Caring Inquiry: The Esthetic Process in the Way of Compassion," suggested that caring inquiry is a unique method of presence and dialogue. Phenomenology, hermeneutics, and esthetic knowing were explored as creative methodologies to study caring as the human and critical mode of being and becoming in nursing.

In closing, I extend a special thank you to the officers and board members of the IAHC, the conference coordinators under the direction of Dean Patricia Starck and Assistant Dean Gwen Sherwood, and all of the participants in the Twelfth Caring Research Conference. We came together for a common purpose and with this publication we have once again told our story for the world and the profession of nursing about care/caring and becoming more human.

A very special word of gratitude goes to the IAHC peer reviewers (listed below), and NLN editors, Sally Barhydt and Allan Graubard, for this publication. The expertise, time, and effort spent in critiquing and editing the contributed papers has provided the reader with the very best in caring scholarship.

IAHC Peer Reviewers

Agnes Aamodt, PhD, RN, Professor Emerita
University of Arizona College of Nursing
2330 W. Wagonwheels
Tucson, AZ 15745

Ann Boykin, PhD, RN
Dean, College of Nursing
Florida Atlantic University
Boca Raton, FL 33431

Joyceen Boyle, PhD, RN
Professor and Chair
Department of Community Nursing
Medical College of Georgia School of Nursing
Augusta, GA 30912

Linda Brown, PhD, RN
Seattle, WA

Kathy Gardner, MSN, RN
Director of Research
Rochester General Hospital
1425 Portland Ave.
Rochester, NY 15610

Nancy O'Connor, PhD
Assistant Professor
Oakland University School of Nursing
Rochester, MI 49309

Doris Riemen, PhD, RN
Director, University of Texas at Tyler School of Nursing
3900 University Blvd.
Tyler, TX 75701

Sister M. Simone Roach, PhD, RN
Coordinator, Mission Education
St. John's Hospital
One Hospital Drive
Lowell, MA 01853

Grace Roessler, PhD, RN
Coordinator, Continuing Education for Health Professionals
Golden West College
Huntington Beach, CA 92647

Phyllis R. Schultz, PhD, RN
Coordinator, Nursing Administration
Community Health Care Systems SM-24
University of Washington School of Nursing
Seattle, WA 98195

Gwen Sherwood, PhD, RN
Assistant Dean for Educational Outreach
University of Texas Health Science Center at Houston School of Nursing
1100 Holcombe Blvd. 5.512
Houston, TX 77030

Sue A. Thomas, EdD, MSN
Professor, Department of Nursing
Sonoma State University
1801 East Cotati Ave.
Rohnert Park, CA 94928

Kathleen L. Valentine, PhD, RN
Director of Nursing Education and Research
The Mary Imogene Bassett Hospital
One Atwell RD
Cooperstown, NY 13326

Delores A. Gaut, PhD, RN

1

Historical Review of the International Association for Human Caring Research Conferences 1978–1990

Delores A. Gaut

The First National Caring Research Conference was convened and hosted by Dr. Madeleine Leininger at the University of Utah in Salt Lake City, April 27–28, 1978. The title of the first conference, "The Phenomena and Nature of Caring," highlighted both the initial and continuing concern of the conference—identifying the philosophical, epistemological, and professional dimensions of caring to advance the body of caring knowledge. The 16 enthusiastic participants underscored the need for an in-depth, think-tank sharing conference designed to explore scholarly ideas about caring and offer support for scholars engaged in caring research. As a result of that first dialogue, the conferences have been directed toward four major goals:

1. Identification of major philosophical, epistemological, and professional dimensions of caring to advance the body of knowledge that constitutes nursing and to help other disciplines use caring knowledge in human relationships.

2. Explication of the nature, scope, and functions of caring and its relationship to nursing care.

1

3. Explication of the major components, processes and patterns of care or caring in relationship to nursing care from a transcultural nursing perspective.

4. Stimulation of nurse scholars to systematically investigate care and caring and to share their findings with other interested colleagues.

Plans were made to continue with yearly national conferences in various demographic regions throughout the United States to stimulate national interest in theoretical, clinical, and research studies related to caring and nursing care. The motto of the group, "Caring is the essence of nursing and the unique and unifying focus of the profession," continues to serve as the key referent and symbolic guide for the future.

The second conference sponsored by Dr. Leininger at the University of Utah, March 22–23, 1979, focused on the study of caring phenomena in cultures and practice settings and involved scholars from anthropology as well as nursing. The focus of the conference, "Analysis of Caring Behaviors and Processes," invited research studies of caring phenomena in cultures and practice settings and involved scholars from anthropology as well as nursing.

The third national conference, "Characteristics and Classification of Caring Phenomena," also held at the University of Utah, under the guidance of Dr. Leininger, focused specifically on classifying the various types of caring phenomena. Some 32 participants attempted to address specific questions related to the classification of the concept:

1. What caring constructs must be included or excluded from a taxonomy?

2. By what criteria is such a judgement made?

3. What are identifying caring taxons?

The proceedings of the first three national caring conferences were published in 1981 and edited by Dr. Leininger, *Caring: An Essential Human Need*, C. B. Slack. Inc. This book was republished by Wayne State University Press in 1989.

The fourth conference moved to Statesboro, Georgia, at the invitation of Em Olivia Bevis. The focus, "Caring and Education: Teaching, Curriculum and Clinical Perspectives," engaged 30 participants. Presenters shared three days of southern hospitality and discussed caring as a concept, caring research, caring as a curriculum model, and caring as a process for interacting with patients and learners.

The fifth national conference, "Discovering Caring in its Fullest Dimensions," moved to Wayne State University in Detroit, Michigan, hosted by the College of Nursing March 17–19, 1981. The purpose of this conference was to assist nurses to critically explore the many embedded concepts, meanings, functions, and relationships within the construct of caring, and explore in-depth the meaning of caring in a health-illness perspective. Many of the papers presented identified both the cultural and professional folk meanings and functions of caring among various cultural groups such as Guatemalans, urban Latinos, southern-rural and anglo-white Americans, and Appalachians.

The sixth conference, held at the University of Texas-Tyler, April 6–8, 1983, was hosted by Dr. Doris Riemen, Dean of the School of Nursing, with this focus: "Caring Theory and Research." Presenters specifically addressed caring theory and research methods in an attempt to assist participants to develop and critique quantitative and qualitative research methods and their applicability to the development of caring theory. Participants engaged in discussions to identify critical issues and problems related to the study of caring, the utilization of caring literature and research studies in teaching and practice, and the comparative analysis of methodological techniques.

The seventh conference went east to Philadelphia, Pennsylvania, April 11–13, 1984. Hosted by LaSalle College of Nursing and Dr. Zane Wolf, the theme maintained focus on the development of caring theory and research methodology with special emphasis on qualitative methodologies such as ethnoscience, phenomenology, and historical research. In 1984, papers from these four conferences appeared in *Care: The Essence of Nursing and Health*, as edited by Dr. Leininger and published by C. B. Slack. In 1988, this book was reprinted by Wayne State University Press.

The eighth caring conference, April 27–29, 1986, "The Caring of Nursing: A Proud Heritage Building New Dimensions," was organized by Dr. Patricia Larson as an invitational conference for those nurse scholars who demonstrated a commitment to the study of caring as evidenced by published and presented papers specific to caring and nursing. The invitation was also extended to doctoral students at the candidate level currently working with faculty involved in research on caring. Sixty-five persons participated in the conference. The conference was planned as a time to review work that had been done in the area of caring and to determine what the future directions of study might be. The site chosen for this working conference was a retreat setting (Vallambrosia) 40 miles south of San Francisco, California. A number of the scholars presented new and refreshing approaches as they discussed communicating human care through esthetics.

The group returned to Vallambrosia Center for the ninth conference April 26–28, 1987, hosted once again by the California members, Dr. Patricia Larson and Dr. Sue A. Thomas. The conference, "Ethics and Morality of Caring," was designed as an opportunity for clinicians and scholars to engage in collegial exchange about issues related to the caring concept in nursing. Ethical and moral perspectives of caring were discussed with implications for nursing practice and advancing of caring knowledge. In 1990, papers from this conference appeared in *Ethical and Moral Dimensions of Care,* as edited by Dr. Leininger, and published by Wayne State University Press.

It was at these two California conferences that the idea of charter membership was first proposed as a way to continue support for the research conferences and provide a more established networking system. Charter members contributed a fee and received a certificate, a list of members, and an updated bibliography on caring literature. Dr. Doris J. Riemen, treasurer for the Caring Conferences, organized and provided these services.

At the invitation of Dr. Anne Boykin, Dean of the School of Nursing at Florida Atlantic University, the conference headed south again to Boca Raton, Florida. One hundred participants engaged in three days of sharing, warmth, and support at the May 1–3, 1988, conference entitled, "Caring: A Living Presence." The presenters included both nurses and clergy, and the papers presented discussed spirituality, suffering and caring, intimacy and nursing, and harmonious interconnectedness.

In 1989, the papers from these three conferences appeared in *Care: Discovery and Uses in Clinical and Community Nursing,* as edited by Dr. Leininger and published by Wayne State University Press.

Denver, Colorado, was the site of the eleventh caring conference as hosted by Dr. Jean Watson and the University of Colorado Health Sciences Center School of Nursing in 1989. The theme, "The Caring Imperative in Education," drew the largest number of participants to date. Some 250 nurses, including visitors and presenters from Sweden, Norway, and Canada, shared in discussing essential issues to be addressed in the educational setting related to caring. The esthetic experiences provided throughout the conference highlighted a variety of caring expressions. The curriculum models presented evidenced the growing interest in caring as a major concept in nursing education and caring practices in the teaching–learning enterprise. In 1990, the papers from this conference appeared in *The Caring Imperative In Education,* as edited by Dr. Leininger and Dr. Watson, and published by the National League for Nursing.

The Denver conference demonstrated the growing interest in the National Caring Research Conferences. The participation had grown from an informal, enthusiastic group of 16 to a cast of 100s including nurse researchers, educators, and practitioners not only from the United States but internationally as well. Our Canadian friends first suggested we think about organizing into a formal association to provide an avenue for continued financial support and membership. The board members, who had been guiding the progress of the caring conferences over the past ten years, formalized the group as the International Association of Human Caring (IAHC) and the charter members voted on the by-laws, officers, and board members at the Twelfth Caring Research Conference in Houston, Texas, 1990.

Between April 27-29, 1990, the International Association for Human Caring and the University of Texas Health Science Center at Houston, School of Nursing, under the direction of Dean Patricia L. Starck and Assistant Dean Gwen Sherwood, co-sponsored the Twelfth Annual Caring Research Conference entitled "Caring: The Compassionate Healer—A Call to Consciousness." The papers presented examined the role of the nurse as the compassionate healer, analyzed the impact of caring expressions in the lives of patients, and advanced scholarly inquiry in caring through formal and informal dialogue. There were 152 participants with 30 states represented and international participants from Canada, Iceland, New Zealand, and Taiwan. This publication, *Caring: The Compassionate Healer*, as edited by Dr. Gaut and Dr. Leininger includes representative papers from this conference, and independently submitted scholarly papers on caring.

As the IAHC looks forward to our first international conference in Australia and projected conferences in Canada, Scotland, and the Scandinavian and Nordic countries, we are even more aware of the Association's responsibility to continue to focus on caring as a global agenda. In all of our endeavors, we have tried to come together as fellow sojourners, united in our purpose and goal, and renewed in the human phenomenon of caring. We share our united consciousness and through that effort create a universal, global force for transformation. We have written and will continue to write a story for the world, and especially for the profession of nursing.

2

The Call to Consciousness: Compassion in Today's Health World

Sister M. Simone Roach

INTRODUCTION

The health world is a microcosm of the anxieties and questions that now preoccupy humanity (Tillard, 1981). The birth of new life and the process of healing as well as the stark and cruel impact of violence and injustice are well known to the health world. Also known to their world, our world, are the many ethical problems that reveal to us, in particularly acute ways, a crisis of moral conscience.

The world in which we live is crying out for compassion, meaning, tenderness, and love. This "call to consciousness," then, is a call to get in touch with this world, particularly with its woundeds; to acknowledge the dissolution of part of its life and history, and to gain hope from the great possibilities for change. We experience our humanity in trial and turmoil, but also, in heroic gestures, we find ourselves seeking definition and new expression. Although success in an evolving new world order is a possibility, it cannot come about unless it is grounded in human compassion.

The nursing profession, by its very nature and mandate, has the great privilege of standing in the health care world with a tradition of love and

7

caring. Its power for moving the world toward a more humane resolution of the crises it now experiences is both formidable and reassuring. By profession we draw forth, in ourselves and in others, the capacity every human being has to care. As never before, we have the opportunity to model this infinite power of love.

Available literature provides for systematic documentation of the contribution of nursing scholarship and research on the human phenomenon of caring and on its centrality in nursing. In this paper, time or space does not permit giving credit to those of you who have and continue to add to this body of knowledge. Perhaps I can best indicate my respect and recognition by calling attention to a work by Janet Smerke (1989) in which many if not most of these works have been cited.

To fulfill the terms of the discussion as I have noted them, I will focus this paper on the following three points: (1) my own reflections on an ontology of caring and its ontical manifestations; (2) a brief overview of some historical developments which have shaped our western culture; and (3) the impact of these developments on today's health world.

AN ONTOLOGY OF CARING AND ITS ONTICAL EXPRESSION

When reflecting on caring, it is helpful to consider the following categories of questions. Ontology raises the question: What is the "being" of caring? What is caring in itself? Anthropology raises the question: What does it mean to be a caring person? Onticology, referring to the study of some entity in relation to other entities, focuses on caring attributes and on the question: What is a nurse doing when he or she is caring? Epistemology addresses ways in which caring is or can be known; pedagogy is concerned with ways in which caring is learned and taught. The following reflections are concerned primarily with an ontology of caring and its ontical manifestations.

From an ontological perspective, caring can be conceptualized as the human mode of being. You and I care, not because we are nurses, but because we are human beings. Caring is the expression of our humanity, and it is essential to our development and fulfillment as human beings. While our capacity to care is somewhat fragile and must be nourished and called forth, and while it may be repressed or suppressed, this capacity yet is nearly indestructible (May, 1969).

As a human mode of being, caring is not unique *to* nursing in the sense that it distinguishes nursing from other professions. Rather, caring is, unique *in* nursing as the concept which subsumes all the attributes descriptive of nursing as a human, helping discipline. Nursing is no more and no less than the professionalization of the human capacity to care through the acquisition and application of the knowledge, attitudes, and skills appropriate to nursing's prescribed roles. As our way of being in the world, caring involves a multiform expression. To understand this multiform expression of caring further, I have found it helpful to categorize it under *five* C's—Compassion, Competence, Confidence, Conscience and Commitment. Here is an example to illustrate.

While preparing these reflections, I was reminded of an experience in the Nursing Division of St. Boniface General Hospital involving nursing directors and staff in the nursing office. It was our anticipation of the birth of a first baby of one of our colleagues with a pregnancy complicated by all the components of high risk. During this very precious and precarious stage in her life and that of her baby, however, she was supported by all the components of human caring—*compassion*, experienced in the manner in which we entered into her experience, each according to one's unique relationships with her and her husband; *competence*, reflected in the medical and nursing expertise in a tertiary care center of high reputation; *confidence* in the people and in the system, and in the moral-ethical bonds reflecting the *conscience* operating within this system; and, finally, *commitment* attested to by ongoing, scrupulous monitoring and support so that the new mother's health could be maintained at an optimum level, and so her special gift would come to fruition. Ashley was delivered by Caesarean section on January 31, 1990. As a Nursing Division, we celebrated the miracle of new life.

You and I experience care both personally and professionally, but we inevitably face the paradox that caring is often more obvious by its absence than by its presence in human affairs. We need to reflect on this paradox and on factors which so frequently contribute to the tension between what is hoped for and what remains: the reality we must deal with. What, then, are some of the historical realities and present trends that are part of the problem?

AN HISTORICAL CONTEXT

Within our lifetimes, planetary events of great magnitude have occurred with unparalleled frequency; changes in world geographic boundaries are unfolding before our eyes. As we experience the past and the future melting into the present, a call to consciousness moves us to look beyond the headlines in the press and television, and to ponder the movements of the past several centuries which have shaped our present culture. These movements embrace a record of glorious achievements; they also include dark and destructive moments in our history. In acknowledging and responding to the latter, we know and affirm that hope resides in the tremendous gift but also in the horrendous burden of our human capacity for change. The challenge to change is the crucial test facing all of us as world citizens today. This is why the theme you have chosen for this Twelfth Annual Caring Conference is so prophetic and urgent; and I believe it is no mere coincidence it was your choice for 1990, the beginning of the last decade of this millennium.

According to a critique by the eminent sociologist, Pitirim Sorokin (1964), this century, with its explosions of wars, revolutions, crime, and violence, is "the bloodiest of all the preceding twenty-five centuries of Greco-Roman and Western history" (p. 24). This is so despite the fact we have made leaps in scientific discovery more astounding than in any previous age of our history, and promise to advance with even greater speed in the future. In communications technology alone, we have created the conditions of possibility for everyone on this planet to live as neighbors.

Sorokin, who makes the above observation, provides a comprehensive critique of what he describes as the "crisis of our age." In a work of this title, he notes:

> Contrary to the optimistic diagnosis, the present crisis is not ordinary but extraordinary. It is not merely an economic or political maladjustment, but involves simultaneously almost the whole of Western culture and society, in all their main sectors. It is a crisis in their art and science, philosophy and religion, law and morals, manners and mores; in the forms of social, political, and economic organization, including the nature of the family and marriage—in brief, it is a crisis involving almost the whole way of life, thought, and conduct of Western society. More precisely, it consists in a disintegration of a fundamental form of Western culture and society dominant for the last four centuries. (1942, p. 16-17)

The crisis referred to by Sorokin involves the dissolution of the sensate culture, a form which emerged in Western civilization at the end of the twelfth century and became dominant after the fifteenth, supplanting the preceding religious or ideational form which prevailed during the medieval period from about the seventh to the thirteenth century (1964, p. 18). One dominant characteristic of the sensate culture is reflected in a naturalistic humanism, which claims the physical is all there is and that the only way of knowing reality is through the method of the empirical sciences. Reality is what we can taste, see, smell, feel, touch, and manipulate. In the sensate view, if the metaphysical or supernatural exists, we have no way of knowing it.

The sensate culture, of which you and I are beneficiaries, ushered in the marvelous achievements in science and technology and major breakthroughs in research that have been our great sources of prosperity and freedom. However, this same sensate culture has created as well our capacity for global and ecological destruction. Like the ideational culture which preceded it, our sensate culture is in crisis because it has become reductionist. Where the previous ideational culture failed because it became exclusively *supersensory*, ours is failing because it has become exclusively *sensory*. Sensate culture has materialized human life and values.

Among the great thinkers who challenge and raise the consciousness of the modern world, Sorokin is not alone. In his famous Commencement Address delivered at Harvard University, June 8, 1978, Aleksandr Solzhenitsyn referred to the decline of Western civilization and raised this question: "How did the West decline from its triumphal march to its present disability?" Solzhenitsyn notes, as the West reacted to a despotic repression of our physical nature in favor of our spiritual nature, it then recoiled from the spirit and embraced all that is material, as if life did not have any meaning beyond physical well being and the accumulation of material goods. This he refers to as "the calamity of an autonomous, irreligious humanistic consciousness" (p. 49). He continues:

> We have placed too much hope in politics and social reforms, only to find out that we were being deprived of our most precious possession: our spiritual life. It is trampled by the party mob in the East, by the commercial one in the West. This is the essence of the crisis: the split in the world is less terrifying than the similarity of the disease afflicting its main sections. (p. 49)

Both spiritual exhaustion and moral poverty comprise the disease Solzhenitsyn claimed to be infecting the capitalist West and the Socialist blocs. His diagnosis confirms Sorokin's observation that, in the nineteenth century, the creativity of the sensate culture began to show signs of fatigue and disintegration. Andrei Sakharov, whom I had the great pleasure to see and hear in person when he came to accept an International Award at the St. Boniface Hospital Research Foundation in 1989, has repeatedly expressed these concerns and has done so at great cost to his own life and well being and that of his family.

This brief discussion certainly would not be complete without reference to another seminal study which mirrors, in more specific ways, American society today. I refer to a source which I suspect is familiar to you, the book *Habits of the Heart*, by Bellah et al. (1986). Based on and borrowing from the 1830s analysis of the French social philosopher Alexis de Tocqueville in his *Democracy in America*, the authors use the term "habits of the heart" in the same sense as de Tocqueville, who used it to refer to the mores which helped shape the character of the American people. He singled out family life, religious traditions, participation in local politics "as helping to create the kind of person who could sustain a connection to a wider political community and thus ultimately support the maintenance of free institutions" (1986, p. viii). The central problem of the book by Bellah et al.

> *concerns the American individualism that Tocqueville described with a mixture of admiration and anxiety. It seems to us that it is individualism, and not equality, as Tocqueville thought, that has marched inexorably through our history. We are concerned that this individualism may have grown cancerous — that it may be destroying those social integuments that Tocqueville saw as moderating its more destructive potentialities, that it may be threatening the survival of freedom itself."* (viii)

This is the world the profession of nursing shapes and is shaped by. The challenge for an integral world and for an integral professional culture was perhaps never so real and never so urgent as it is at this moment in our history: we are literally dealing within timeframes of weeks and months, not decades or centuries. Our values, our commitments, and our choices today determine the future of nursing, and the future of nursing is intimately connected to the future of humanity. It is an exciting privilege, but also a demanding challenge to be part of humanity's journey during this unique and perhaps perilous time as we approach the third millennium.

COMPASSION IN TODAY'S HEALTH WORLD

What do these reflections have to do with a "Call to Consciousness: Compassion in Today's Health World"? A prior question we might ask is, What does it mean for you and for me to be involved in this health world? As one contemplative writer responds to this question,

> *To be involved in the health world therefore no longer means integrating oneself into a clearly demarcated sphere, dispensing with all responsibility but that of a lively professional conscience. On the contrary, it means standing at one of the crossroads of our world's problems and joining up there with man [men and women] no longer fleeing from suffering and death but anxiously seeking for fullness of life.* (Tillard, 1981, p. 17)

The health world is the meeting point of the anxieties and major questions now preoccupying humanity—questions which carry a special poignancy and resonance because they bring us into direct contact with life, with birth, suffering and pain, with recovery, and death. This world mirrors all the miracles of new life and healing, of love and reconciliation; and, in stark and cruel ways, it also mirrors the impact of injustice and violence.

While you and I share in the wonderful life-giving moments of our professional and personal involvements, we are all too familiar with the injustices of preferential treatment, the hardships of poverty and old age, the abuse of children and of the elderly, exploitation of women and the violence of pornography. We experience the conflicts of power-seeking and competition within our own professional relationships; when we deny our call to servanthood, "compassion becomes spiritual stardom" and turns into its opposite— competition (McNeill et al., 1982, p. 38). In the words of Tillard (1981), we see this health world mirroring violence, "not a violence beneath its brutal mask, but a violence often suffered so unconsciously that it becomes, so to speak, the daily companion of modern life." (p. 19)

The health world is one of the mainstreams of today's ethical problems, and Tillard (1981) makes the observation "our society is shaken by a crisis of moral conscience" (p. 23). As we face the ultimate questions of life and death, this crisis is experienced on a daily basis. We note it in the observations of a Professor of Law at University of California Law School at Berkeley who claims we are living in the first society in human history where an elite in society, where a society, through its leadership, supports abortion as a good. The leadership to which he refers is the media, the federal judiciary, great philanthropies, and doctors, particularly doctors associated with teaching hospitals (Noonan, 1980, p. 99). We see it in the debate on euthanasia where motives to kill out of mercy are justified under the name of "beneficence." We encounter this crisis in the daily press, and as I am writing this paper, in the announcement that a woman has conceived a child to provide a suitable donor for her daughter with leukemia. Her husband reversed a vasectomy to make this possible.

The health world of which you and I are a part and within which we play significant roles is a world in need of a soul, in need of tenderness and love. It is a world crying for compassion, asking us, according to Nouwen (1980), to go

> where it hurts, to enter into the places of pain, to share the brokenness, fear, confusion, and anguish. Compassion challenges us to cry out with those in misery, to mourn with those who suffer loneliness, to weep with those in tears. Compassion requires us to be weak with the weak, vulnerable with the vulnerable and powerless with the powerless. Compassion means full immersion in the condition of being human. (p. 3)

The health world is a world searching for the spiritual, the transcendent, a world in search of meaning. It calls us to consciousness of the values that shape our thinking and mold our decisions; to examine the fallacies of a reductionist humanism which denies anything beyond the physical and the empirical, and to question the inadequacies of a mechanistic view of science that reduces all phenomena to matter and chemical analysis.

As I was preparing my reflections for this conference, I was conscious of the world-shaking events in Europe, South Africa, South America, and the participation of other countries of the world in shaping their futures. One concern kept surfacing in my thoughts: If the new world is to be built on political power and economic stability alone, are we as a human race in danger of repeating the historical blunders and atrocities of the past? The "signs of the times" indicate this need not be so. The great "implosions," as they are called, have an element of spiritual transformation that can create a world more glorious than we have ever known. But it is helpful to remember implosions create vacuums, and this is essentially what experience of crisis is—"one world has died; another is powerless to be born . . . . The experience of it is the experience of crisis or dilemma, of being condemned to the anxious space between the no-longer and the not-yet" (Rowe, 1980, p. 13).

These reflections are not intended to communicate an apocalyptic message of gloom and doom. To do so would fail to take into account that which is very much within our reach and within our range of choice. In his 1964 work, Sorokin discusses an integral culture—a blend of the ideational and the sensory which we have experienced in the past, perhaps only for short moments of time, but now have the freedom to create for the future. In 1964, Sorokin already had noted the changes and tendencies toward a cultural "mixed type" involving the capitalist and socialist bloc countries. His concluding comment, in its prophetic wisdom, is the challenge and the crisis we now face.

> *If a peaceful and unimpeded government of today's mixed type is given a real chance, there is hardly any doubt that eventually it will grow into a unified type of a magnificent integral order in both countries [United States and Russia] as well as in the whole universe. Each country will build this new order in its own variation and each variation is likely to be nobler, more creative, and better than most of the previous sociocultural orders in human history. Viewed in this light, this convergence is a hopeful symptom and a healthy process. As such it can be heartily welcomed by all who really care about man, culture, and all the immortal values created by man on this planet. (p. 130)*

Each day nurses are saving lives, and moment by moment, in ways not always documented, you and I provide a presence that is enabling for others, that empowers patients, families, colleagues, and staff. We do this because we enter into the experiences of others, because we reverence human life and human values. Theorizing about compassion in the abstract, however, is not sufficient: We must exercise moral imagination. Through moral imagination we are able to picture the suffering of others and to suffer with—"cum patior"—to enter into the heart of that universal mystery of compassion which is central to the Judeo-Christian and other traditions. It is suffering with those who suffer, expressed in Buddhism as *karuna*. Is this not what compassion is about?

I introduced my reflections by sharing a personal experience of the *five C's* of caring. May I conclude by sharing a beautiful exemplar from a study by Fenton (1987) that describes a nurse's belief in the value of a patient, and in the need to make the death of a particular man a caring event.

> *I looked after a man whose address was the bus shack outside of the Mall Hotel. I sat there and I held his hand and I watched him die, through a whole night. It was Saturday night and I thought to myself, this is a very strange job I have. You know, you're looking outside and seeing the stars and you know people are out and it's Saturday night and I'm sitting there holding a man's hand . . . because he's going to die. He has nobody to be with him when he dies. It made me feel very rewarded. I felt in some ways pleased that I could be with him. He didn't have to be alone. He opened his eyes occasionally and he knew someone was there and I held his hand.* (p. 195)

This exemplar demonstrates compassion, an entering into the experience of the other; care, not determined by class or worth or social status, but grounded in the nurse's sense of another human person in need of someone. It demonstrates the fulfillment experienced by the nurse through human caring, through reaching out to the other, to investing herself in the other. The value the nurse perceived in this man, whose address was the bus shack, was rooted in her perception of his humanity. I do not know the nurse who shared this touching experience, but I sometimes wonder if she was not also struck by a sense of mystery—that the dignity of this human being whose hand she held during his dying was grounded also in his being made in the image of God.

Human care has been a focus of special interest to philosophers, theologians, poets, and artists for centuries, and it is the focus of our deliberations over the next two days. The following ancient Roman myth is perhaps a fitting conclusion to my reflections this afternoon.

Once when "care" was crossing a river, she saw some clay; she thoughtfully took up a piece and began to shape it. While she was meditating on what she had made, Jupiter came by. "Care" asked him to give it spirit, and this he gladly granted. But when she wanted her name to be bestowed upon it, he forbade this, and demanded that it be given his name instead. While "Care" and Jupiter were disputing, Earth arose and desired that her own name be conferred on the creature, since she had furnished it with part of her body. They asked Saturn to be their arbiter, and he made the following decision, which seemed a just one: "Since you, Jupiter, have given its spirit, you shall receive that spirit at its death; and since you, Earth, have given its body, you shall receive its body. But since 'Care' first shaped this creature, she shall possess it as long as it lives. And because there is now a dispute among you as to its name, let it be called 'homo', for it is made out of humus."

According to this fable, while we live on earth, our truest name is "care." That is to say, we essentially are care: *care is our human mode of being.* When we cease to care, we cease to be human.

SELECTED BIBLIOGRAPHY

Bellah, R. N., Madsen, R., Sullivan, W. M., Swidler, A., & Tipton, S. M. (1986). *Habits of the heart*. New York: Harper and Row.

Dawson, C. (1960). American and the secularization of modern culture. *The Smith History Lecture*. Houston: University of St. Thomas.

Dubay, T. (1973). *Caring: A biblical theology of community*. Denville, NJ: Dimension Books.

Fenton, M. T. (1987). *Ethical issues in critical care: A perceptual study of nurses' attitudes, beliefs and ability to cope*. Unpublished master's thesis, University of Manitoba, Winnipeg, Canada.

Fox, M. (1979). *A spirituality named compassion*. Minneapolis: Winston Press.

Frankl, V. W. (1963). *Man's search for meaning: An introduction to logotherapy*. New York: Washington Square Press.

Gaylin, W. (1979). *Caring*. New York: Alfred Knopf.

Hauerwas, S. (1986). *Suffering presence*. Notre Dame, IN: University of Notre Dame Press.

Kelsey, M. (1981). *Caring*. New York: Paulist Press.

Lobel, E. (1976). *My mind on trial*. New York: Harcourt Brace Jovanovich.

May, R. (1969). *Love and will*. New York: W. W. Horton, pp. 284–285.

Mayeroff, M. (1971). *On caring*. New York: Harper & Row, Perennial Library.

Milford, J. E. (1985). Omnicide and the sanity of compassion. *The Christian Century, 102*, 93–94.

McNeill, D. P., Morrison, D. S., & Nouwen, H. J. M. (1982). *Compassion: A reflection on the christian life.* New York: Darton, Longman & Todd.

Noonan, J. T. (1980). Is abortion a private choice? In: *The new technologies of birth and death: Medical, legal and moral dimensions.* St. Louis: The Pope John Center.

Nouwen, H. J. M. (1972). *The wounded healer.* New York: Doubleday.

Nouwen. (1974). *Out of solitude.* Notre Dame, IN: Ave Maria Press.

Nouwen. (1977). Compassion in a callous world. *Sojourners. 6*, 15–18.

Richards, M. (1964). *Centering.* Middleton, CT: Wesleyan University Press.

Reich, W. T. (1989). Speaking of suffering: A moral account of compassion. *Soundings, 72*, 83–108.

Roach, M. S. (1984). *Caring: The human mode of being, implications for nursing.* Toronto: Faculty of Nursing, University of Toronto.

Roach, M. S. (1987). *The human act of caring: A blueprint for the health professions.* Ottawa: Canadian Hospital Association.

Rowe, S. C. (1980). *Living beyond crisis: Essays on discovery and being in the world.* New York: Pilgrim Press.

Smerke, J. M. (1989). *Interdisciplinary guide to the literature on human caring.* New York: National League for Nursing.

Solzhenitsyn, A. (1978). *A world split apart.* New York: Harper and Row.

Sorokin, P. A. (1942). *The crisis of our age.* New York: E. P. Dutton.

Sorokin, P. A. (1964). *The basic trends of our times.* New Haven, CT: College and University Press.

Thera, P. (1964). *The Buddha's ancient path.* London: Rider.

Tillard, J. M. R. (1981). The health world. A place for the following of Christ. *Lumen Vitae, 36*, 7–44.

Vanier, J. (1986). Called to compassion. *The Other Side, 22*, 14–17.

3

The Contexts of Caring: Conscience and Consciousness

Mary-Therese Dombeck

INTRODUCTION

Conscience has been described as a state of moral awareness; a compass directing one's behavior according to the moral fitness of things (Roach, 1984). In this paper, I will present a theoretical framework for describing and analyzing perspectives on moral awareness in the contexts of caring encounters.

This paper was inspired by a larger research project entitled "Dream-Telling and Professional Personhood." In that study, I assumed that, as dream-telling engages imaginal and thematic aspects of human communication, it also facilitates personal story-telling at different levels. Even when the dream is alleged to be insignificant and unrelated to the dreamer, when told to another the dream becomes a contextually communicated personal story. An experienced dream is a way of being with oneself; a told dream is a way of telling about oneself, and of being with another. I learned much by asking professional persons, nurses among them, to tell their own dreams, and the dreams of persons they were caring for. The descriptions of clinical situations and narratives told in this paper come from participant observation experiences and interviews conducted during the course of that study.

However, first, I have chosen two of my own dreams, which I had while working on this paper to introduce these preliminary remarks. The dreams expressed for me two common perplexing situations and ethical dilemmas faced by nurses in their practice.

First Dream

I am in a foreign country. There is a woman who looks like Emily (a woman I care for in my psychotherapy nursing practice). She lives in this deserted territory. It is a sort of valley—like a depression in the landscape with caves and blocks of rock. When I arrive in that place I see that there has been an act of sabotage. I am trying to speak with her, but we are not understanding each other because of language. I'm supposed to find out who or what was responsible for the danger and how to help. I wonder if she is in danger, I want to help her; but she is very elusive; she keeps disappearing behind the rocks, and occasionally reappearing.

Second Dream

Eve (a client) is supposed to come to the clinic at 11 o'clock. She comes to my house before 11 o'clock. My home (in the dream) is just across the street from the clinic. She comes into my living room and says she is hungry. I offer her a peanut butter sandwich but she wants a bologna sandwich. I say emphatically: "but I only have peanut butter." I feel frustrated. At one point I even go to bed determined to sleep for a while in spite of the commotion, knowing that she is waiting outside my bedroom door.

Both dreams express in image and story encounters between a *nursing person* and a *nursed person* or more broadly speaking, one caring and one cared for (Noddings, 1984). The actions in the dream occur in a context which includes the *experienced environment*, the *personhood* of the actors, and their apprehension and awareness of their experience or their *self-reflexivity*.

The *experienced environment* of each dream represents contrasting situations. In the first dream I see myself in foreign territory; more specifically I am in the territory of the nursed person. In the second dream she is in my house. I perceive her to be invading my own territory. In the first dream I am the pursuer. I want to help her; I am supposed to be involved in her safety, but she keeps evading and eluding me. In the second dream, it is the nursed person who pursues. She will not allow me to ignore her. She compels a response. I have to escape temporarily just to get a nap.

In terms of our *personhood*, in both dreams we are in a reciprocal relationship with designated rights and obligations toward each other. In the first dream I know what I am supposed to do, but the task is difficult because of a language barrier. Moreover, she is evasive and elusive. She uses her environment to hide from me. In the second dream, she knows exactly what she wants, but, first, I don't have it to give, and, second, there is a hint in the dream (suggested by a play of the word "bologna"/baloney, and my emphatic answer about peanut butter) that I think what I want to give her is better for her than what she wants.

In terms of *self-reflexivity*, each dream offers to me the opportunity to ponder the experience of my encounter with the nursed person. I notice my experience. I ponder the quality of my attentiveness to another, and in so doing I am attentive to myself. My thesis is that the quality of my capacity to attend to another increases as I engage freely in my own experience. Thus conscience is contingent on, and indeed inseparable from, consciousness.

CONTEXT

These two dreams are provided as introductory exemplars of two different contexts in which caring encounters occur. In any nursing encounter the *nursing person* and the *nursed person* approach each other as actors in a moral universe; their actions are contextualized by their respective experienced environments, their personhood, and their self-reflexivity (see Figure 3–1).

The practice of nursing is diverse and adaptable to different eras and different settings, implying a flexible consistency in time and space. Whether the nurse sits with, does with, does for, or does on behalf of another, he or she has an opportunity and a responsibility to foster health by providing a caring presence in contexts of human vulnerability.

A context is not simply a setting. It also includes the social roles, the social history, the relationships, the moral rules, the personal histories, and each actor's awareness of himself or herself and of the other in that particular context. It involves temporal, spatial, normative, perceptual, and noetic aspects of experience.

The distinction between the concepts of *person* and *self* is helpful in understanding the complexities of context. It is not uncommon for people in Western societies to speak of person and self as synonyms. We are also prone, on the one hand, to describe ourselves subjectively as individualities and psychological entities or personalities, and, on the other hand, to postulate an objective reality outside of our own perception of it.

For this reason, I distinguish *person* as a member of society, invested with social capacities and responsibilities to be the author of actions considered to

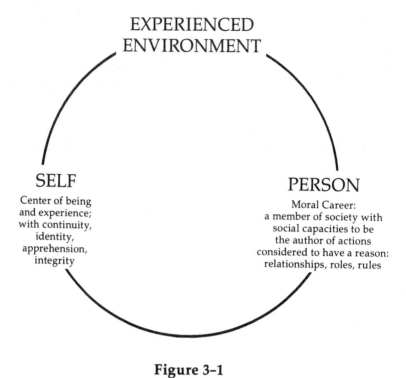

EXPERIENCED
ENVIRONMENT

SELF
Center of being
and experience;
with continuity,
identity,
apprehension,
integrity

PERSON
Moral Career:
a member of society with
social capacities to be
the author of actions
considered to have a reason:
relationships, roles, rules

Figure 3-1

have a reason (Mauss, 1938; Beck, 1965; Krader, 1968; Fortes, 1973; Harris, 1989) from *self* as center of being and experience (Cooley, 1964; Mead, 1934; Goffman, 1959; Fogelson, 1982). Both person and self are part of the experienced contextual environment. Thus it is neither accurate to see ourselves exclusively as biological and psychological entities without any reference to our social personhood, nor is it accurate to perceive our social and physical environment as external to ourselves and apart from our own experience of it (Benner & Wrubel, 1989; Csordas, 1990).

The distinction I propose between *person* and *self* is experientially nonexistent. The person *is* the self and the self *is* the person. This assumption is made explicit by the fact that the person/self is continuous with the experienced environment. It both creates it, and is created by it. This is the *context* of the situation.

It was my dialogue with nurses in a seminar on ethical issues which convinced me that the distinction between person and self was useful. We were discussing the ethical dilemmas that were created by blindly imposing moral

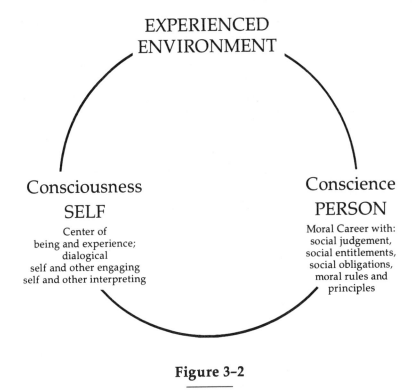

Figure 3-2

principles and rules out of the context of a situation. One of the nurses said thoughtfully, "A nurse, when alone, has a lot of conscience to contend with." When we examined this statement and others like it, we realized it was important to remember to think contextually, while resisting the temptation to resort to subjectivism and relativism by proposing that the rules are different for each person. It is also important to remember that this very conundrum is part of our context in Western societies. It is our emic reality, and one that we, as nurses, have had to contend with constantly. Even though as human beings we experience ourselves as whole, and as nurses we want to practice holistically, as persons in Western or industrialized societies we find ourselves with persons and systems, including our very thoughts and linguistic processes, that make us engage in dualistic, mechanistic, objectivistic or subjectivistic ways of seeing others and ourselves. While we proclaim our holism, we often experience ourselves as fragmented in our own contexts.

Therefore, for the purposes of this discussion, I propose that our *conscience* is derived from our social personhood, while our *consciousness* is experienced in engaging our self. Moreover, both of these concepts are contingent on, and indeed, continuous with, each other. However, distinguishing the two gives us a way, on the one hand, to be less ethrocentric, by neglecting our own and other cultural and social influences on our caring encounters, and, on the other hand, to overcome the disjunction of mind and body by acknowledging that we are dialogical, self-engaging, self-interpreting human beings, who also engage other selves in caring encounters (see Figure 3–2).

PERSON: COMPREHENDER OF CONSCIENCE

The concept of person has been used extensively in nursing literature. It appears in nursing philosophy statements and in nursing models as one of the important phenomena of interest for professional nurses. *Person* also has been studied extensively in psychological, sociological, anthropological, and humanistic literatures.

Although, I cannot, in the scope of this paper, offer a complete summary of the literature on this important concept, I will summarize ways in which the concept has been used in connection with conscience.

Person in this context connotes moral agency (Mauss, 1938; Fortes, 1973).[1] It describes someone who because of his or her social judgment, social entitlements, social position, social history, and social relationships is deemed capable of doing the right thing. Children acquire their personhood gradually as they acquire the capacity for social judgment.[2] Similarly, in this context people can lose some of their personhood when they lose their social entitlements (as with offenders of criminal or civil laws and norms), or their social judgment (as with persons acknowledged to be cognitively incompetent). In all societies personhood is given and taken away according to special criteria (Harris, 1989).[3] We all know of individuals who have been depersonalized (Goffman, 1961), that is, who, because of their social standing, or cognitive incompetence, are not yet, or are no longer deemed capable of social and moral agency.

When nurses become professional persons their duties and entitlements are added to their social obligations and capacities. They are deemed capable and are expected not only to have good social judgment like other persons but also to have good clinical judgment. Moreover, they are expected to be, and they expect themselves to be, caring and compassionate. The question "What is expected of me?" involves the nurse's comprehension of all of these issues related to his or her personhood even before encounter with patients begins. Sometimes different expectations conflict with each other and bring the nurse into personal conflict or into conflict with other persons.[4]

An exemplar will illustrate this point. When I asked nurses to tell me their dreams about themselves and their patients, one of the experienced psychiatric nurses in a community mental health center told me of a dilemma she experienced. Patients were telling her nightmares about incestuous situations and other violent abuse. By talking to these patients, she discovered that the abuse was actual in their waking life, and they were also dreaming about it. (These are psychiatric patients who are often assumed to have strange dreams and fantasies.) It was hard for her to convince her physician colleagues that besides having the dreams the patient had also, in fact, been abused in waking life. She says:

> You're taught (as a nurse) that you have to look for the spiritual, the family, the financial; so these are things that always sort of come natural to me. An example is, because I'm a nurse, I started early a long time ago hearing a lot of stuff about incest and sexual abuse before it was fashionable, you know. They would dream about it and then talk about it. The physicians at first didn't want to believe me. They said that didn't happen very much. "Come on! They're making this up." Well, I had a student who wanted to do a project, so we gathered some data, and we found a lot of incest. I also ask questions about religion and how this has played as a positive or negative issue in some of the people's illness. Those are some of the things I have to question. The holistics thing, that you have to see this person as a whole, but it was hard at first to do this here.

In this case, the nurse's relationship with her patients, her capacity to understand and to believe her patients, created disbelief and skepticism in her relationship with physician colleagues. She must choose either to believe the physician's theory that there is no basis in fact to the patient's story or to believe her patients. This is not easy to do when patients, as these, have a psychiatric diagnosis. Moreover, she must make decisions on the basis of her own values and conclusions. This is such a common happening that we do not think of it as an ethical dilemma. The answer to the questions "What am I expected to do?" and "What is expected of me?" would be easily come by if one could simply follow rules, but in the context of her personhood she has to care enough for her patients to be faithful to them, and yet be professionally competent enough to discern whether her patients are engaging in fantasy, telling metaphorical truths, or telling factual truths. Like the nurse in the ethics seminar mentioned earlier, she could have said "a nurse, when alone, has a lot of conscience to contend with." The nurse has to engage, not only the person she nurses, but also her *self* (see Figure 3-3).

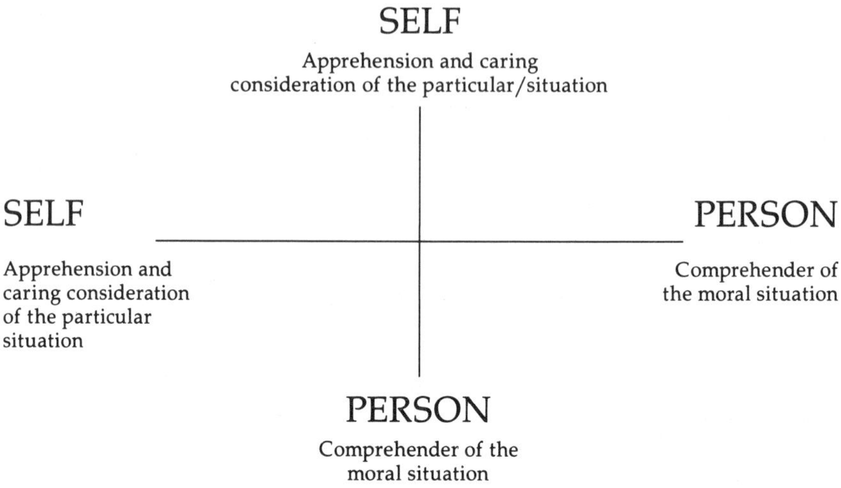

SELF
Apprehension and caring
consideration of the particular/situation

SELF   PERSON

Apprehension and   Comprehender of
caring consideration   the moral situation
of the particular
situation

PERSON
Comprehender of the
moral situation

Figure 3-3
Contexts of Caring Encounters

SELF: APPREHENDER OF CONSCIOUSNESS

The concept of *self* has been studied in relationship to the nursed person and the nursing person, usually in terms of self-concept (Peplau, 1952), self-care (Orem, 1971), self-actualization (Schlotfeldt, 1975), an emerging open energy field (Rogers, 1986), a spiritual ideal capable of transpersonal caring (Watson, 1985). The self has also been studied extensively in psychoanalysis (Goldberg, 1982), psychology (Hartman, 1950; Jung, 1951; Erikson, 1963; Piaget, 1962, 1966), self-psychology (Kohut, 1977; Goldberg, 1980), social psychology (Cooley, 1922, 1964; Mead, 1959; Goffman, 1959, 1961), anthropology (Hallowell, 1954, 1966; Le Vine, 1980; Fogelson, 1982; Crapanzano, 1982; Lienhardt, 1985), philosophy (Buber, 1970; Heidegger, 1962; Husserl, 1964; Taylor, 1985), and theology (Tillich, 1952; Van Kaam, 1982).

In studies and theories of the *self*, including those done in the nursing disciplines, a persistent problem arises from a previously described dilemma: whether to consider the self always and only an experiencing subject, or whether to consider the self a duality, where in one aspect, the self is *subject*, author and chooser of behavior, and in other aspects, an empirical *object* in a material world; an object factually and socially real to others and to oneself.

This dilemma has perpetuated a dualism of objectivism versus subjectivism in the practice and research communities, including nursing. The history of Western philosophy and scholarship has included many different dualisms during different eras. My own ethnographic research among American psychotherapists suggests an ethos of perceived dualities and disjunctions between mind and body, inner life and outer life, private life and public life, and waking life and dreaming life. Sometimes, even when persons profess holism they experience incongruities, disjunctions, and dilemmas (Dombeck, 1991). The mind/body duality is not only a predominant tenet of certain Western philosophies but also a contemporary cultural ethos and a popular emic understanding of Western persons, so it can neither be completely ignored nor completely accepted in our research methodologies. It must not remain an unrecognized assumption.

I propose that the concepts of *person* and *self* can help us understand, express, and investigate caring encounters in general, and nursing situations in particular. For the self is the center of being and experience in persons. Our experience as selves is also dialogic. We communicate not only with others but also we are in constant contact with our selves. Our bodily knowledge, our fantasies, our dreams are all ways of being with our selves. Our contact with our selves is both immediate and mediated by our personhood and the collective cultural and historical wisdom or folly of the social groups to which we belong. We apprehend ourselves to be continuous with ourselves and identical with ourselves (these experiences come to us in our apprehension of time and space). We attend to what we care about including and especially the self.

When two persons encounter each other, each has an understanding of the context in terms of what is socially expected (calling forth aspects of *personhood*), as well as in terms of one's particular apprehension of the situation (which the *self* experiences). The context becomes constellated according to how each one comprehends and apprehends the total situation. Sometimes, each can have different expectations of the situation; at other times, although there is agreement on what is expected, each brings to the particular context different experiences and unique ways of being in the situation.

In certain contexts in life the encounter constellates primarily about aspects of personhood. For example, in brief encounters with bank tellers, or at ticket counters at airports, the interaction is conducted primarily in terms of social role and function. The persons involved have little opportunity for access into each other's experience. Yet even in those encounters, nuances of the self are expressed by nonverbal demeanor.

There are other contexts where each person's unique self is the main aspect of the encounter. Examples of this are to be found in contexts of transition and danger when persons are compelled to engage themselves in essential and intense ways. Many nursing contexts are ones in which transition, danger and intimacy are present.

CONTEXTS OF CARING

The *person* is he or she who comprehends the moral aspects of an encounter. Formal and informal educational systems in all societies are instituted with the goals of teaching designated members of groups to understand social situations.[5] Furthermore, with regard to the health professional educational systems, the whole process is a painstaking attempt to take a person who already understands the social situation and teach him or her to also understand the clinical situation in all of its moral significance.

An encounter between a nursing person and a nursed person in terms of personhood is defined as one of *comprehension* relating to what ought, or ought not, to occur, and to what is expected of a professional nurse. In this context the moral questions are: "What ought I to do?" "What is expected of me?" and, for the nursed person, "What can I expect from this nurse?" These questions exist even before the nursed person and nursing person encounter each other. For novices these important questions are in the foreground; for nurses who have experienced similar situations in the past the question is assumed and assimilated as part of the nurse's sense of identity, continuity, and personal integrity (Benner, 1984) (see Figure 3-4).

But for the novice or the expert, as soon as the encounter begins the context is constellated. The person does not just comprehend. Much more is apprehended than what is expected or what ought to occur. There are personal memories, bodily sensations and knowledge, emotions, intentions, thoughts, and, of course, anxieties (apprehension) to name a few. There is awareness of one's awareness (like looking at a mirror image of oneself looking at the mirror). In these contexts, there is always an apprehension that one has grasped more than one can comprehend, and that, at the same time, one knows less than one wants to know about the situation. It is this situation which arouses *concern*, as the question changes from, "What is expected of me?" to "Who am I to you?" Moreover, the latter question is embedded in the ontological reality of "Who am I?" "How am I?" It is as I engage myself in this way that I become a self, and become able to encounter another, not as a rule-designated object but as another "myself."

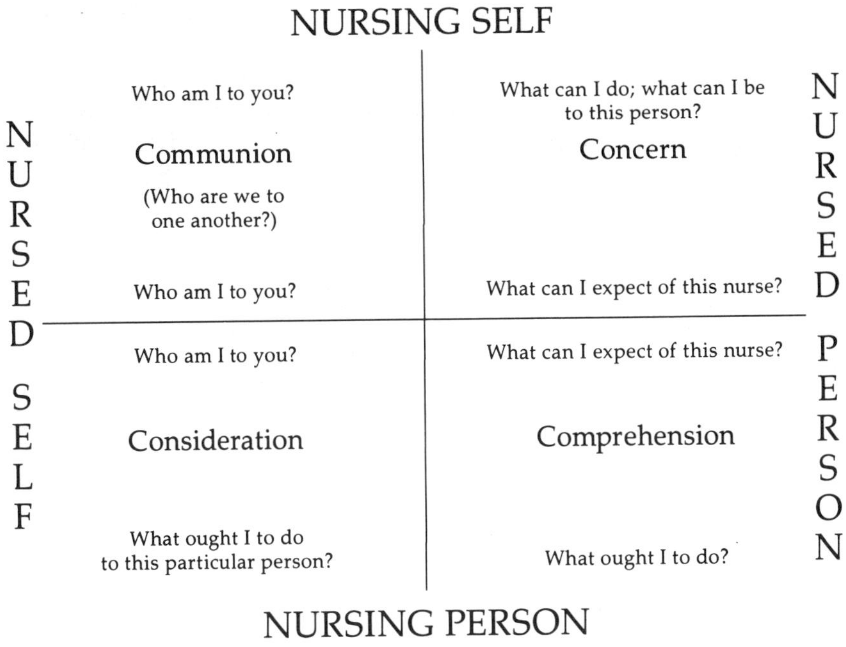

NURSING SELF

	Who am I to you? **Communion** (Who are we to one another?) Who am I to you?	What can I do; what can I be to this person? **Concern** What can I expect of this nurse?	N U R S E D
N U R S E D S E L F	Who am I to you? **Consideration** What ought I to do to this particular person?	What can I expect of this nurse? **Comprehension** What ought I to do?	**P E R S O N**

NURSING PERSON

Figure 3–4

Concern

It is in such contexts as described that the nurse engages the nursed person with concern. A concerned nurse gives caring attention to the particular situation not only because he or she is a professional *person* but also and especially because her experienced *self*, with all its understandings, misunderstandings, and other apprehensions are now engaged. Now the nursed person matters at a different level. He or she has entered my intimate experienced world, my feelings, and even my dreams and fantasies (Dombeck, in press). It is no longer a matter just of what I am supposed to do, but also of who I am, and who I am willing to become.

Many nurses have told me their thoughts, feelings, concerns, and dreams of persons they were caring for. Typically, in these situations the nursed persons have no understanding initially or at any time that they are engaged with such concern; examples are pre-verbal children, rebellious adolescents, comatose patients, depressed patients, or indeed any patients in situations of transition and danger who are unable to express themselves to the nurse in that particular environment.

The following example will illustrate the quality of concern I have described. This narrative was told by a clinical nurse specialist who was responsible for a population of chronically mentally ill patients. It is remarkably like many I have heard, and somewhat like my own dream of the elusive patient in the foreign country. She says of her patient:

> I dreamed about him when he disappeared. He sort of disappears for awhile you know . . . there was no way of getting in touch with him at all, because he didn't have a phone and he wasn't working, and so my dream was that he was going to kill himself.
>
> What did you think of that? I asked.
>
> Well, I thought it was—I think I woke up and I was pretty angry with him, and I guess I was pretty angry with the system that I'm in, because I had asked to have a special review of this man. And it seemed to be dragging on and on and I guess I was just so scared that this man was going to kill himself—you can have a special review when you have a case you don't feel is going right and you sense that there is a kind of danger or something. I wanted some validation that I had done all I could do.

This same nurse told me that she had gone out to the clients' homes, and that she believed the current structure of psychotherapy was totally inadequate for the patients she saw whose environment was different from others in the health care system. It was this man who aroused her concern.

Consideration

There is another type of situation that is frequent in nursing. Sometimes the nurse attempts to approach the nursed person through aspects of personhood, primarily in terms of what ought to be done, and what is expected, but the nursed person challenges, pursues, importunes, and otherwise compels a more personally involved response from the nurse. It is as though the nursed person were saying: "It is I we are talking about. I am unique. You will neither overlook me, nor treat me like you do everyone else." These are not only the persons who make many demands, but also persons who because of their intensity, the danger they are in, or because of the quality of their engagement of themselves seem to similarly engage the nurse. These persons refuse to take on the traditional sick role and insist on challenging erroneous assumptions about them. They demonstrate more vulnerability, strength, or courage than we expect. They usually challenge us to mobilize resources we do not have, or do not know we have. They call us to engage our own self more intimately and intensely. They help us to bring to the particular situation a quality of caring consideration which is higher than we had anticipated.

The following example from another mental health clinical specialist who learned from her client how angry she could become will illustrate. She says:

> He was a very irritating kind of person very passive aggressive. I just ignored the fact of how angry I was becoming. And one night I had this dream about him, in which he was standing outside my house at my home. He wanted to come in, finally in the dream I said, "No, I'm not going to let you in, enough is enough, go away or I'll call the police." And I remember I was so furious that I kind of woke up.
>
> What did you think of that dream? I asked.
>
> Well, at first I was kind of appalled that I wouldn't let somebody who wanted to come into my house, and I was a little scared that I was so angry. This was the last straw this person was not going to invade my life. At that time I woke up.
>
> It [the experience] tuned me right into what I was feeling in the dream. When I looked at it I stopped. I said: Whoa! You really are angry with this guy and you need to do something different in therapy to make it tolerable, cause you're going to end up doing something terrible to him. I felt that way. I was a kind of self-awareness. I did not tell him the dream. I said to him that I was getting more angry and frustrated because we weren't getting anywhere. I said it nicely she added laughing.

In contexts of caring consideration it is the nursed person who helps us engage ourselves more authentically. They compel us to grow and become more.

Communion

When in a nursing situation the nursed person and the nursing person engage themselves and each other freely, the context is defined as communion. There is a meeting of selves in which the moral question is not only "What can we expect from one another?" but also and especially "Who are we to one another?"

This context does not necessarily describe situations where everything is successful, or where there is agreement. Rather, it is a context in which participants share their experience freely with one another, where each stands before the other in their essential humanity. In these contexts there is a possibility of learning compassion.

The context of communion is to be distinguished from situations of enmeshed relationships or of self-absorption. In enmeshed relationship, the persons are compulsively attached to each other in one sense, but in other aspects, they have left themselves behind. In this situation, both the self and the other are used as objects of attachment. In self-absorption, you treat yourself as an object of attachment.[6] When you are, in large degree, unavailable to yourself, you cannot attend freely to another.[7] The nurse who discovered that she was angry with her client was consequently able to share more of herself with him. She moved from a position of comprehending that she must be responsible toward her client to a position of caring enough about him to engage her own anger and to share her frustration with him.

SUMMARY AND IMPLICATIONS

In this paper, I have maintained a distinction between *person* and *self* in order to describe and analyze contexts of caring in nursing encounters. As the nursed person's perspectives are examined in light of the nurse's capacity to engage his or her own experience, four contextual categories emerge: comprehension, consideration, concern, and communion.

Such concepts can help us describe and analyze many situations in clinical nursing and in nursing education. The following paragraphs describe several of the possibilities for future research:

It is important to study in which contexts in nursing *personhood* and *selfhood* are enhanced and when they are diminished.

Diminishment of personhood leads to *depersonalization* which describes a condition of loss of agency and helplessness in a world where others are in control. This can happen to the nursed person and to the nursing person. When nurses are placed in contexts where they experience lack of agency and authority in their practice settings (even when they attempt to engage others with concern and compassion), they can start to feel and become depersonalized.

Diminishment of self leads to *dehumanization*, which describes a loss of contact with one's own experience. Rules and relationships are oppressive or inflexible and the participants experience meaninglessness. For example, how long can nurses be in daily situations of administering painful procedures to patients without experiencing dehumanization? The same question can be asked of nurses at all levels in hierarchies, and in all relationships, for example, nursing instructors with students, nurse administrators with staff nurses, faculty in academic institutions, and staff nurses with each other. Depersonalization and dehumanization eventually lead to one another.

Another significant question to explore could be this: In which of the four contexts defined above does the nurse experience most satisfaction, most dissatisfaction, and the condition we call burnout?

We live in a world, a society, and a profession where depersonalization and dehumanization are the plight of many. How can personhood and selfhood be enhanced or even restored in our hospitals, clinics, classrooms, and academic institutions? I propose that investigations of the contexts of caring can help us explore, discover, describe, and analyze these questions.

NOTES

[1] Mauss (1938) analyzed the concepts of *person* and *self* in a historical perspective. He traced the evolution of Western notions of person as historically emerging from the concept of role, and mask to that of the social person who is conscious, independent, autonomous, free, and responsible. He postulated that the birth of moral consciousness is the originator of conscience, which is an aspect progressively added to the concept of legal and moral uprightness in Western history. This evolution continues until a sense of self (*moi*) develops. The self is a psychological person, an individual possessed of metaphysical and moral value.

There are many problems with Mauss's analysis. Namely, he presents an evolutionistic and ethnocentric view of what he perceives to be a qualitative difference between traditional societies and Western societies in their understanding of themselves, and second, he does not address the Cartesian dualism explicitly. The advantages of Mauss' work are, first, that he suggests that all *persons* have a sense of corporal morality as well as a sense of themselves and, second, he looks at persons within their own contexts. Another advantage of this theory is that it provides recognition of our own context. No matter how insistently we protest the dualistic dilemmas in which we find ourselves, however, we must admit that they have affected and influenced us and the persons we work with and care for. We have a tendency to reproduce them.

[2] Children who break social rules and laws are treated differently than adults who commit similar actions in the same society. However, people who are deemed to have lost their senses are also expected not to be capable of understanding social contexts, and are also treated differently from sensible adults when they have behaved improperly or broken the law. Social blunders, immoral conduct, absurd behavior, or illegal actions always call into question the judgmental capacities of the person. The question here usually concerns whether the person is knowingly in breech of social conventions and norms, or whether the person is lacking in

judgmental capacities. In the case of social blunders, persons are expected to receive further education in social skills or social sophistication. In the case of immoral or illegal actions, persons are expected to apologize, make amends, or pay their dues to society as the case may be. In the cases when persons are deemed incapable by reason of insanity, they can obtain legal defense, but at the price of being relegated to positions of marginal personhood.

[3]Harris (1989) also understands the notion of person to be universal and sees persons as agents in society, having moral careers with socially ascribed capacities and responsibilities: namely judgmental capacities, social entitlement capacities, and mystical capacities. These capacities and responsibilities are not merely role expectations added to the person. They are part of one's own personhood in a moral universe. Unfortunately, Harris fails to deal with the subjective experiential aspect of each context he discusses.

[4]Each role acquired brings its own set of rights, relationships, and obligations; these become a part of the context, not only in themselves but in the personal story of the particular actor. Moral dilemmas are created for the person when two roles have conflicting moral expectations.

[5]One example of a test of this capacity is the Mental Status Exam which is designed to test cognitive, emotional, and social competence. It is expected to demonstrate whether persons are capable of comprehending the consequences of their actions or of their failures to act. Most clinicians have discovered that such tests, because of their focus on social judgment within a particular cultural context, are ethnocentric when administered out of context for the persons tested.

[6]In monotheistic theological language, self-absorption or absorption in another as an object would constitute idolatry, because the dialogue between the created self and the creator is absent. In the language of Eastern systems of spirituality, self-absorption and absorption in another would constitute unbalanced attachment and illusion.

[7]Peplau's work on interpersonal anxiety demonstrates the importance, on the one hand, of the individual apprehending enough of his or her context for learning to occur, and on the other hand, of controlling high levels of anxiety that can make it impossible to learn or communicate dialogically.

REFERENCES

Beck, L. W. (1965). Agent, actor, spectator and critic. *The Monist, 14,* 167–182.
Benner, P. (1984). *From novice to expert: Excellence and power in clinical nursing practice.* Menlo Park, CA: Addison-Wesley.
Benner, P., & Wrubel, J. (1989). *The primacy of caring: stress and coping in health and illness.* Menlo Park, CA: Addison-Wesley.

Buber, M. (1970). *I and thou*. (Walter Kaufman, Trans.). New York: Charles Scribner's and Sons.

Cooley, G. H. (1964, 1922). *Human nature and the social order*. New York: Schocken.

Crapanzano, V. (1982). The self, the third and desire. In *Psychosocial theories of the self* (pp. 179–206). New York: Plenum.

Csordas, T. J. (1990). Embodiment as a paradigm for anthropology. *Ethos, 18*(1), 5–47.

Dombeck, M. T. B. (in press). *Dream-telling and professional personhood: The contexts of dream telling and dream interpretation among American psychotherapists*.

Erikson, E. (1963). *Childhood and society*, (2nd ed.). New York: Norton.

Fogelson, R. D. (1982). Person, self, and identity: Some anthropological retrospects, circumspects, and prospects. In *Psychosocial theories of the self* (pp. 67–109). New York: Plenum.

Fortes, M. (1973). On the concept of person among the Tallensi. In G. Dieterlin (Ed.), *La notion de personne en Afrique noire*. Paris: Editions de la Recherche Scientifique.

Goffman, E. (1959). *The presentation of self in everyday life*. Garden City, NY: Doubleday.

Goffman, E. (1961). *Asylums: Essays on the social situation of mental patients and other intimates*. Garden City, NY: Anchor Books.

Goldberg, A. (1980). *Advances in self psychology*. New York: International Universities Press.

Goldberg, A. (1982). The self of psychoanalysis. In *Psychosocial theories of the self* (pp. 3–21). New York: Plenum.

Hallowell, A. I. (1954). The self and its behavioral environment. In *Culture and experience* (pp. 75–110). Philadelphia: University of Pennsylvania Press.

Hallowell, A. I. (1966). The role of dreams in Ojibwa culture. In G. E. Grunebaum & R. Callois (Eds.), *The dream in human society*. Berkeley: University of California Press.

Harris, G. G. (1989). Concepts of individual, self, and person in description and analysis. *American Anthropologist, 91*(3), 600–612.

Hartman, H. (1950). Comments on the psychoanalytic theory of the ego. In *Essays on ego psychology* (pp. 182–206). New York: International Universities Press.

Heidegger, M. (1962). *Being and time*. (M. J. Robinson, Ed.). New York: Harper & Row.

Husserl, E. (1964). *The idea of phenomenology*. (A. W. Nakhikan G., Trans.). The Hague: Nijhoff.

Jung, C. G. (1951; 1971). *Aion*. Vol. 9. (H. G. Baynes, Trans.). Princeton: Bollingen/ Princeton University Press.

Kohut, H. (1971). *The analysis of the self*. New York: International Universities Press.

Krader, L. (1968). Person, ego, human spirit in Marcel Mauss: Comments. *The Psychoanalytic Review, 55*(3), 482–490.

Le Vine, R. A. (1982). The self and its development in an African society: A preliminary analysis. In *Psychosocial theories of the self*. New York: Plenum.

Lienhardt, (1985). Some African representations of self. In M. Carrithers, S. Collins, & S. Lukes (Eds.), *The category of the person: Anthropology, philosophy, history* (pp. 141–155). Cambridge: Cambridge University Press.

Mauss, M. Une categorie de l'esprit human: La notion de personne. *Journal of the Anthropological Institute, 68,* 262–281.

Mead, G. H. (1959). Mind, self and society. In A. Strauss (Ed.), *The social psychology of George Herbert Mead* (3rd ed.). Chicago: University of Chicago Press.

Noddings, N. (1984). *Caring: A feminine approach to ethics & moral education.* Berkeley: University of California Press.

Orem, D. E. (1971). *Nursing: Concepts of practice.* New York: McGraw-Hill.

Peplau, P. E. (1952). *Interpersonal relations in nursing.* New York: Putnam.

Piaget, J. (1962). *Play, dreams, and imitation in childhood.* London: Routledge and Kegan Paul.

Piaget, J., & Inhelder, B. (1966). *The psychology of the child.* New York: Basic Books.

Roach, S. (1984). *Caring. The human mode of being: Implications for nursing.* Perspectives in Caring. Monograph, 1, Toronto Faculty of Nursing, University of Toronto.

Rogers, M. E. (1986). Science of unitary human beings. In V. M. Malinski (Ed.), *Explorations on Martha Roger's science of unitary human beings* (pp. 3–8). Norwalk, CT: Appleton-Century-Crofts.

Schlotfeldt, R. M. (1975). Research in nursing and research training for nurses: Retrospect and prospect. *Nursing Research, 24,* 117–183.

Sullivan, H. S. (1953). *The interpersonal theory of psychiatry.* New York: Norton.

Taylor, C. (1985). *The concept of person in human agency and language: Philosophical papers 1* (pp. 97–114). Cambridge: Cambridge University Press.

Tillich, P. (1952). *The courage to be.* New Haven and London: Yale University Press.

van Kaam, A. (1982). *The emergent self.* Denville, NJ: Dimension Books.

Watson, J. (1985). *Nursing. Human science and human care: A theory of nursing.* Norwalk CT: Appleton-Century-Crofts.

4

Five Basic Modes of Being with Another

Sigridur Halldorsdottir

When the weak and the orphaned
are deprived of justice
all the foundations of the earth
are shaken.

Ps. 82.3–5

Leininger (1988) maintains that caring is the essence of humanity, and that it is essential for human growth and survival. She contends that care is one of the most powerful and elusive aspects of our health and identity and must be the central focus of nursing and the helping and healing professions. Similarly, Roach (1988) claims that care is the basic constitutive phenomenon of human existence and thus ontological in that it constitutes man as man. She points out that all existentials used to describe Dasein's self have their central locus in care. Roach states, "When we do not care, we lose our being and care is the way back to being. Care is primordial, the source of action and is not reducible to specific actions" (1987, p. 15).

Although Roach (1984) claims that caring is the human mode of being, she wonders how convincing the view is that caring is the natural expression of what is authentically human when there is so much evidence of lack of caring, both within our personal experiences as well as in the society around us. Roach points out that we live in an age where violence is commonplace and where atrocities are committed against individuals and communities everywhere. To compound the effect of such violence on the broader social body, many incidents enter our living rooms through the press, radio, and television often as quickly as they occur.

As a result, modes of being with another in our world involve both caring and uncaring dimensions. What, then, are the basic modes of being with another? By analyzing two of my own studies on clients' (patients' and students') perceptions of caring and uncaring encounters (Halldorsdottir, 1989, 1990), as well as related literature, I have determined that there are five basic modes of being with another: life-giving (biogenic), life-sustaining (bioactive), life-neutral (biopassive), life-restraining (biostatic), and life-destroying (biocidic) (see Figure 4-1 and Table 4-1).

In this chapter, I will describe the five basic modes of being with another through examples of caring and uncaring encounters in hospitals as experienced by former patients, my coresearchers in the former study (Halldorsdottir, 1988). The phenomenological perspective of qualitative research theory guided the methodological approach to the studies analyzed, involving the use of theoretical sampling, intensive unstructured interviews, and constant comparative analysis.

Nine former patients participated in the former study and data were collected through 18 in-depth, open-ended interviews. Nine former nursing students participated in the latter study and data were collected through 16 in-depth, open-ended interviews. In both studies, interviews were tape-recorded and transcribed verbatim for each participant.

The excerpts used from the former study will be referred to as "modes of being with a patient," and for the sake of clarity, the feminine will be utilized in reference to the nurse, the masculine in reference to the coresearcher/patient/client. In the text, however, "nurse" and "coresearcher/patient/client" can

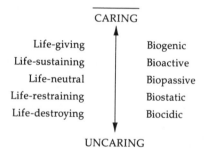

Figure 4-1
The Caring/Uncaring Dimension or Continuum

Table 4-1
Five Basic Modes of Being with Another

Life-destroying (biocidic) mode of being with another is a mode where one depersonalizes the other, destroys joy of life, and increases the other's vulnerability. It causes distress and despair, and hurts and deforms the other. It is transference of negative energy or darkness.

Life-restraining (biostatic) mode of being with another is a mode where one is insensitive or indifferent to the other and detached from the true center of the other. It causes discouragement and develops uneasiness in the other. It negatively affects existing life in the other.

Life-neutral (biopassive) mode of being with another is a mode where one does not affect life in the other.

Life-sustaining (bioactive) mode of being with another is a mode where one acknowledges the personhood of the other, supports, encourages, and reassures the other. It gives the other security and comfort. It positively affects life in the other.

Life-giving (biogenic) mode of being with another is a mode where one affirms the personhood of the other by connecting with the true center of the other in a life-giving way. It relieves the vulnerability of the other and makes the other stronger and enhances growth, restores, reforms, and potentiates learning and healing.

---

refer to both males and females. Evidence from literature, that has a bearing on this matter, also will be given.

The *life-destroying*, or *biocidic, mode* is the most inhumane mode of being with another in the list as given and is represented by violence in all its forms. It means hurting, harming, or deforming the other. This destructive mode manifests in numerous ways: making people dependent or fostering infantilism; being threatening; involving manipulation, coercion, hatred, aggression, and humiliation; involving various kinds of abuse; and often involving an evident lust for power, followed by dominance and depersonalization of the other. Hardheartedness or coldheartedness also may be present here. This mode of being with another most often changes the other to the worse, the harm done depending on the other's strength to endure. It involves the transference of negative energy or darkness to the other. It is the frost the human flower has a hard time enduring without loosing its luster, its petals, its leaves, its very life.

In many respects, the history of humankind is not a positive affirmation of the sanctity of human life as Roach (1987) has rightly pointed out. There seems to be no end to how destructive and brutal the human being can be. Roach also argues that perhaps the greatest threat against human life in our age lies in the erosion of sensitivity toward its value, particularly where the taking of human life becomes part of everyday experience. Roach claims that the public at large has become less and less sensitive to all overt killings— genocide, fratricide, homicide, suicide, and feticide.

As described, the *life-destroying*, or *biocidic*, *mode of being with a patient* is the most severe form of indifference to the patient as a person, involves harshness and inhumanity, and is characterized by various forms of inhumane attitudes. Although I will not tell their entire stories here, four out of the nine coresearchers in the study under discussion had a biocidic experience. Of those four coresearchers, three asked me whether I had seen "One Flew over the Cuckoo's Nest" and claimed that their nurse was very much like nurse Rachet as portrayed in that film. None of the coresearchers knew each other.

While all coresearchers held a unanimous perception that uncaring encounters with nurses were very discouraging and distressing experiences for them as patients, their reactions to such encounters were many sided. Several major themes were identified in their accounts: *initial puzzlement and disbelief*, which is followed by *anger and resentment*. Because of the patient's vulnerable circumstances, however, the patient is most often unable to act out feelings of anger and resentment, and these strong negative feelings seem to develop into *despair and helplessness*.

Being uncared for in a dependent situation develops feelings of impotence, a sense of loss, and a sense of having been betrayed by those counted on for caring. If on top of that the patient is treated by the nurse as if somewhat less than human, the patient's feelings soon develop into feelings of *alienation and identity loss*. The patient feels he has no value as a person, that he is indeed less than a person: "a side of beef," "an object," or "a machine." Furthermore, experiencing uncaring increases the patient's own feelings of *vulnerability* within the hospital setting.

Numerous coresearchers alluded to the threat of dehumanization within today's hospitals. It was their unanimous perception that they felt vulnerable and in need of caring when they were in the hospital. Some suggested this makes patients more sensitive to caring and uncaring. One such former patient stated:

> I would expect that people being ill makes them vulnerable, so that when they have an uncaring transaction, like someone treats them rudely, they are more deeply wounded in that circumstance than if they were healthy and walking the street and someone on the corner said something stupid or insulting. I mean that they can shrug off and ignore, but here they are sick and in need, and probably feel weak in spirit, and weak in body, and so it hits home harder, any such transaction hurts them more.

Other coresearchers related that they perceived uncaring as a transference of negative energy that affected their well being and delayed or even prevented their recovery. This perceived *negative effect on well being and healing* is illustrated time and again in their accounts. Furthermore, it was their unanimous perception that the uncaring encounters made such an indelible impression on them, and had a longer lasting effect than caring encounters, that they tended to be both *acid edged and memorable experiences.*

Some coresearchers referred to the "memories of uncaring encounters" as scars, and although they seem to be trying to understand or make sense of the experience they are most often still angry, and even have nightmares about the nurses perceived to be uncaring. Some coresearchers identified how the uncaring experience prompted them to think about ultimate realities vis-a-vis death, affected their view of the hospital, and how it continued to even dictate their decisions within the health care system today.

Although most coresearchers had tried to forgive the uncaring nurse, some coresearchers related that that was probably more a result of forgetfulness than forgiveness. These coresearchers sometimes expressed a longing to return and confront the uncaring nurse, if, for nothing more, than to relieve themselves of their anger. At the same time, however, they realized that the nurses perceived to be uncaring were probably unaware of their influences on the patients and would, therefore, not recognize their stories.

Hildegard of Bingen, a remarkable twelfth-century abbess, scientist, artist, poet, musician, and mystic, talks about the dryness of carelessness and injustice. She claims that dryness and coldness together make hardness of heart and that drying up destroys our creative powers, marking the end of all good works, and the beginning of laziness and carelessness. She maintains that if we lack an infusion of heavenly dew we will be turned into dryness and our souls will waste away. From Hildegard's point of view, the ultimate uncaring occurs when we become cold and hardened to injustice. Hildegard (1985) wrote to one churchman: "When a person loses the freshness of God's power, he is transformed into the dryness of carelessness. He lacks the juice and greenness of good works and the energies of his heart are sapped away" (p. 64).

The *life-restraining,* or *biostatic, mode* of being with another involves negatively affecting life in the other by restricting or disturbing the energy already existent in the other. It means being insensitive or indifferent to the other, causes discouragement, and develops uneasiness in the other. It often involves imposing one's own will upon the other, dominating and controlling the other. It sometimes appears as fault-finding, anger, blaming, accusing, and being unfriendly. It is that very coldness and strong wind the human flower has a hard time enduring.

The *life-restraining,* or *biostatic, mode of being with a patient* involves the patient feeling strongly that the nurse doesn't care and is blind to his feelings by way of negative feedback from nurse to patient. Here, the nurse often treats the patient as a nuisance, that is, if it weren't for the patient the nurse's life would be a lot easier. The patient starts to feel that he is bothering the nurse when asking for help, and finds the nurse often cold and unkind, and the nurse's presence destructive in some way. This nurse approach is partly illustrated in the following accounts.

> The second one [uncaring nurse] was cold, and I can at least give her that much because I interacted with her enough. The first one, I would just say I was . . . what?, I don't know, a piece of dust on the floor, I mean, I can't, I was a bother . . . The people in that room were just beds, that's all, you know, beds. She had prescriptions, she had a checklist of what she had to do, you know, your heart, etc., and that's all it was, for everybody, not just for me, you know.

> I had experiences of being in another ward for three days, and there was a tremendous high percentage of noncaring nurses. Actually, this is a nice description saying noncaring nurses, they were completely like . . . cold . . . cold human beings, like computers. It's like, sometimes I was worried, I was . . . was wondering if they really even noticed that I was there.

Dossey (1982) asserts that a patient-as-object approach to care delivery is destructive because it violates the oneness and wholeness that are necessary for healthy, viable living systems. Similarly, Gadow (1985) has pointed out that in addition to the domination by apparatus and by experts that can accompany the use of technology, patients can be reduced to objects in a more fundamental way than by the use of machines: in the view of the body as a machine. Gadow states, "such reduction occurs because regard for the body exclusively as a scientific object negates the validity of subjective meanings of the person's experience. Those meanings are categorically nonexistent in the scientific object" (p. 36). Furthermore, Gadow (1988) has pointed out that the exercise of power always increases the vulnerability of the one over whom it is exercised, no matter what benevolent purpose the power serves.

The life-neutral, or biopassive, mode of being with another occurs when one is detached from the true center of the other and when there is no effect on the energy or life of the other. This lack of response, interest, and affect derives from inattentiveness or insensitivity to the other. It refers to the lack of a positive or caring approach rather than the presence of something destructive. Although it has no real effect on the life in the other, it sometimes creates a feeling of loneliness, because there is no mutual acknowledgment of personhood, no person-to-person contact. Furthermore, many seem to experience this apathetic inattention not only as lack of care but as noncaring or uncaring.

The fundamental characteristic of the *life-neutral,* or *biopassive, mode of being with a patient* is perceived apathy, which refers to the approach in which the nurse is perceived to be inattentive to patients and their specific needs. The coresearchers emphasized that the nurse seemed to care about the routine, the tasks she was supposed to perform, but not about the patient as a person. The nurse is sometimes perceived by the patient as insensitive, absent-minded, tired, dissatisfied in her job, or lacking in some caring quality, for example, warmth of voice. Furthermore, the coresearchers perceived these nurses as either unwilling, or unable, to connect with, or develop attachment to, the patient. The coresearchers' perceptions of detachment are seen clearly in their accounts. In fact one coresearcher stated, "Aahm . . . the way she looked at you . . . like you are not a part of her world . . . or that she doesn't want to attach—you can feel that there is no emotional attachment there."

Bermejo (1987) asserts that a person is essentially characterized by a necessary openness to another. He contends that a person closed in upon and withdrawn into his or her self, hardly deserves the status of person, for this withdrawal, he argues, goes counter to the very core of man's being, which is clamoring first for an opening, and then, based upon that opening, for a total gift of self to another. Bermejo states, "A rejection of this essential, radical opening and the ensuing personal communion would unavoidably have a crippling effect on the fulness of the human person. A man half open is only half a man" (p. 46).

Hildegard of Bingen (1985) states in one of her many books that too often human actions are weak and lukewarm and emerge from people who are more asleep than awake. She claims that in this way people "make themselves weak and poor who do not wish to be busy about justice or about rubbing out injustice or about paying back their debts." Commitment to justice, she insists, would wake people from their sleep and would put zeal back into their lives and work.

Similarly, Matthew Fox (1985) has pointed out that the theme of spiritual maturity as wakefulness has been expressed in religious literature throughout the world. Hildegard also makes a connection between wisdom as wakefulness and folly as sleepfulness. In the Gospel parable, the wise virgins stayed awake; the foolish fell asleep. In Hildegard's terms, we can never climb the mountain of healing, celebration, justice making, and compassion if we do not care, if we are not committed, if we are indifferent and do not fight injustice.

The *life-sustaining,* or *bioactive, mode* of being with another involves benevolence, good will, genuine kindness and concern, beneficence, and kindheartedness. It is protecting life, relieving suffering, keeping promises, respecting the other, and acknowledging the other's humanhood. Thanking and praising and a contrary dislike of constraining others are involved here. Indeed, there exists the heartfelt wish to do no harm. Comforting, encouraging, consoling, strengthening the other, and continuing to support the energy already present in the other adds other dimensions to the bioactive mode.

The *life-sustaining*, or *bioactive, mode of being with a patient* means that the nurse is skillful, knowledgeable, committed to the provision of personalized care, and knows how to safeguard the personal integrity and dignity of the patient. This special kind of nurse approach, which includes *compassionate competence, genuine concern for the patient as a person, undivided attention when the nurse is with the patient*, and *sober cheerfulness*, is what I call *professional nurse caring* (Halldorsdottir, 1990).

When the nurse succeeded in giving this kind of professional caring, it promoted feelings of trust in patients, which facilitated the development of attachment between patients and nurses. It is precisely this attachment that forms the basis of a life-giving presence where openness and the transference of positive energy, which affects the other in a profound way, predominates.

This *life-giving* or *biogenic mode* of being with another is the truly human mode of being and is represented by healing love. This mode involves loving benevolence, responsiveness, generosity, mercy, and compassion. A truly life-giving presence offers the other interconnectedness and allows for the expansion of the other's consciousness and fosters spiritual freedom. It involves being open to persons and giving life to the very heart of man as a person, creating a relationship of openness and receptivity yet always keeping a creative distance of respect and compassion. The truly life-giving or biogenic presence restores well being and human dignity. It is a transforming personal presence that deeply changes man. For the recipient there is experienced an inrush of compassion, often like a current.

Regarding the *life-giving* or *biogenic mode of being with a patient*, one coresearcher said this about the fundamental difference between caring and uncaring: "I'm not sure how to put it other than 'personal relationship,' the sense is somehow that your spirit and mine have met in the experience. And the whole idea that there is somebody in that hospital who is *with* me, rather than working *on* me."

Another coresearcher explained it this way: "You know, there is that kind of bonding, that kind of feeling of . . . not intimacy but at least *connection*, there has been a connection made with that person, a connection which I could then follow-up on, you know, I would feel free to do so."

From coresearchers' accounts, it is apparent that this bonding or connection also involves a *creative distance of respect and compassion*, a dimension of professional attachment which has to be present in order to keep caring in the professional domain. It is also clear that dimensions in true professional caring depend on the depth of attachment developed. Professional attachment development can be conceptualized as a process involving five phases: *initiating attachment,* or reaching out; *mutual acknowledgment of personhood; acknowledgment of attachment; professional intimacy;* and *negotiation of care* (Halldorsdottir, 1990).

This professional nurse–patient relationship is in many ways unusual. The following two accounts provide poignant illustrations:

> *She fostered a working relationship between the two of us, as I said importantly as equals, and fostered a sense of* independence *for your own growth, your personal growth to the point where you didn't need her in that role anymore.*

> *In most other relationships what you want is some sort of deepening of the ability to communicate or the commitments so that the relationship is ongoing, that is, you want to perpetuate the relationship whereas in nursing and teaching the ideal thing is like parenting, what you want to do is to enable the client to graduate, that is, to leave. The best thing that could happen is that the patient is able enough to stop being a patient. Well, that is a peculiar thing in a relationship, that is, you are hoping for it to stop, for it to be no reason to continue, and then to be able to say goodbye with blessings, so that makes it unusual, I think, as a relationship.*

The coresearchers' accounts illustrate clearly their conceptions of how caring positively influences the patient's ability to recover. Some coresearchers articulated the relief that they sensed when they felt cared for and how that diminished anxiety and gave them time to concentrate on getting better. Some coresearchers actually referred to caring as medicine of sorts. One said,

> *The purpose of the friendliness and the caring is focused on a particular professional activity and a particular very short period in the life of the patient and designed to . . . it's another form of medication of sorts. It's part of the healing, part of the getting the patient better, and it's creating the climate for the patient getting better.*

Some coresearchers emphasized that caring affected healing through the psyche of the person. One said,

> *I think the effect on the psyche of a person is very much a part of the healing, because I believe in treating the whole person, treating them as*

body, mind, and spirit, not just the body alone but the three of them combined, and if their psyche is being damaged or uncared for, then how can their body get well?

It is apparent from the data that the nurse–patient attachment is perceived by the patient as a therapeutic or healing relationship. It seems that professional caring makes healing more profound, more rapid, and better internalized if it is provided, and it definitely makes the patient feel better healed.

In addition, the data makes evident that the patient's reactions to professional caring are quite positive. The professional nurse gets to know the patient as a unique individual and treats that individual accordingly. She communicates to the patient in a way that makes him feel fully accepted as a normal human being, and legitimized as a person and as a patient. This helps the patient to feel all right about himself and his hospital stay. Professional caring also seems to give the patient a sense of hope and optimism, encouragement and reassurance. To feel cared for also gives the patient a sense of security. All this decreases the patient's anxiety, increases the patient's confidence, and positively affects the patient's sense of well being and healing. From coresearchers' accounts, it is evident that they were, and still are, very grateful for their caring encounters; even if the only one, it is a pleasant memory that they carry away from their hospital stay.

Life flows through the life-giving person like a river and there is a transference of positive energy, strengthening, inspiring, comforting, enlightening, and invigorating the other, bringing joy, hope, trust, confidence, and peace. This life-giving presence is greatly edifying for the soul of the other. It involves dynamism, movement, and growth. It is a healing energy of unconditional love. It is the heavenly sunshine and nourishment the human flower needs in order to grow and develop, to learn and to heal.

Examined in theological perspective, this growth-promoting flow of positive energy from the very center of the life-giving person is a "divine" energy of love and light, which has its source in a personal, living, and life-giving God. Fox (1979) contends that compassion is a flow and overflow of the fullest human and divine energies born of an awareness of the interconnectedness of all creatures by reason of their common creator. The preciousness of the human being and the inherent dignity of each person is explained by Archimandrite Sophrony (1977) who states, "When our spirit contemplates in itself the 'image and likeness' of God, it is confronted with the infinite grandeur of man, and not a few of us—the majority, perhaps—are filled with dread at our audacity" (p. 44). He further contends that in the Divine Being the hypostasis constitutes the innermost esoteric principle of Being.

Similarly, in the human being, the hypostasis is the most intrinsic fundamental. As Sophrony states,

> Persona *is the hidden man of the heart, in that which is not corruptible
> . . . which is in the sight of God of great price (I Peter 3.4) —the most
> precious kernel of man's whole being, manifested in his capacity for self-
> knowledge and self-determination; in his possession of creative energy; in
> his talent for cognition not only of the created world but also of the Divine
> world. Consumed with love, man feels himself joined with his beloved God.
> Through this union he knows God, and thus love and cognition merge into
> a single act.* (1977, p. 44)

Again from a theological perspective, those who have gained perfection in caring are called saints. Dumitru Staniloae (1987), a professor of dogmatic theology, provides a closer look at saints. He explains how the gentleness and firmness of the man of God, his power to comfort and his power to incite, his nearness and yet his distance, are all things rooted in the transcendent love of God, which comes close to us in him. Staniloae claims that in the person of the saint, because of his availability, his extreme attention to others, and by the alacrity with which he gives himself to Christ, humanity is healed and renewed. Staniloae states,

> *The saint always radiates a spirit of generosity, of forbearance, of attention
> and willingness to share, without any thought for himself. His warmth
> gives warmth to others and makes them feel they are regaining their
> strength, and lets them experience the joy of not being alone . . . the saint
> immediately creates an atmosphere of friendliness, of kinship, and indeed
> of intimacy between himself and others. In this way he humanizes his
> relationships and leaves on them a mark of genuineness, because he him-
> self has become profoundly human and genuine.* (p. 3)

Staniloae concludes,

> *The saint shows us a human being purified from the dross of all that is
> less than human. In him we see a disfigured and brutalised humanity set
> to rights; a humanity whose restored transparency reveals the limitless
> goodness, the boundless power and compassion of its prototype —God
> incarnate. It is the image of the living and personal absolute Being who
> became man that is re-established in the person of the saint. By being so
> truly human, he has reached a dizzy height of perfection in God, while*

remaining completely at home with men. The saint is one who is engaged in ceaseless, free dialogue with God and with men. His transparency reveals the dawn of the divine eternal light in which human nature is to reach its fulfilment. He is the complete reflection of the humanity of Christ. (p. 7)

This life force, or heavenly sunshine, creates the ideal conditions for the human flower to germinate, sprout, bloom, and bear fruit. It is a positive creative energy through which humanity is healed and renewed.

ONE FAMILY

Father of love
fountain of life and source of light
A dry seed that I am
give that I may dwell in you
and moistened by the dew from heaven
become a fruit of your ever-living love.

Mother of love
venerable rose and queen of tenderness
A hungry child that I am
give that I may rest against your breast
and nourished by your cherishing love
become filled with loving kindness.

Brother of love
divine partner, guide and companion
An unworthy sinner that I am
flood my senses with the light of your love
and sanctified by your gracious brotherliness
give that I may flourish in you
my most dulcet morning.

Sister of love
white lily in the cloister of kindness
A mature woman that I am
with love let me serve you
and in our long white gowns
let us in joy and purity of heart
celebrate our sisterhood.

Sigridur Halldorsdottir

REFERENCES

Bermejo, L. M. (1987). *The spirit of life*. Chicago: Loyola University Press.

Dossey, L. (1982). Care giving and natural systems theory. *Topics in Clinical Nursing*, 3(4), 21–27.

Fox, M. (1979). *A spirituality named compassion*. Minneapolis: Winston Press.

Fox, M. (1985). *Illuminations of Hildegard of Bingen*. Santa Fe, NM: Bear and Company.

Gadow, S. (1985). Nurse and patient: The caring relationship. In A. H. Bishop & J. R. Scudder Jr. (Eds.), *Caring, curing, coping: Nurse, physician, patient relationships*. Alabama: The University of Alabama Press.

Gadow, S. (1988). Covenant without cure: Letting go and holding on in chronic illness. In J. Watson & M. A. Ray (Eds.), *The ethics of care and the ethics of cure: Synthesis in chronicity*. New York: National League for Nursing.

Halldorsdottir, S. (1989). *Caring and uncaring encounters in nursing practice: The patient's perspective*. Paper presented at the International Nursing Research Conference, Nursing Research for Professional Practice, held by Workgroup of European Nurse Researchers (WENR). Frankfurt/Main, September 7, 1989.

Halldorsdottir, S. (1989). The essential structure of a caring and an uncaring encounter with a teacher: The nursing student's perspective. In J. Watson & M. Ray (Eds.), *The caring imperative in education*. New York: National League for Nursing.

Halldorsdottir, S. (1990). *Caring and uncaring encounters in nursing practice: The patient's perspective*. Unpublished manuscript.

Hildegard of Bingen (1985). In M. Fox (Ed.), *Illuminations of Hildegard of Bingen*. Santa Fe, NM: Bear and Company.

Leininger, M. M. (1988). *Caring: An essential human need*. Detroit: Wayne State University Press.

Roach, M. S. (1984). *Caring: The human mode of being, Implications for nursing*. (Perspectives in Caring Monograph 1). Toronto: University of Toronto, Faculty of Nursing.

Roach, M. S. (1987). *The human act of caring: A blueprint for the health professions*. Ottawa, Ontario: Canadian Hospital Associations.

Sophrony, A. (1977). *His life is mine*. (Rosemary Edmonds, Trans.). Crestwood, NY: St. Vladimir's Seminary Press.

Staniloae, D. (1987). Tenderness and holiness. In D. Staniloae, *Prayer and holiness: The icon of man renewed in God*. Fairacres, Oxford: SLG Press.

5

The Energetics of Conscious Caring for the Compassionate Healer

Linda Joseph

"It is a wonderful time to be a nurse," many nurses enthusiastically proclaim. We are making progress in exploring what nursing is, and what we as nurses are about. There is still much to be done in defining our discipline in a way that we can all agree on and convey to others. Yet, there is currently a convergence in the trains of thought of many nursing theorists and philosophers that lends greater clarity and certainty to our profession and its purpose.

This paper provides an overview of some of these trains of thought and how they converge as a meaningful basis for understanding the dynamics of conscious caring. The theoretical works of Martha Rogers, Margaret Newman, Rosemarie Parse, and Jean Watson, significant for their visions of the energetics of compassionate caring, will be discussed briefly. The energetics involved in each of the four ways of knowing in nursing identified by Carper (1986)—empirical, ethical, esthetic, and personal patterns—are also significant and will be discussed briefly. In order for nurses to actualize their potential as compassionate healers, it is imperative that an understanding of the energetics of knowing and caring be a conscious part of the process.

Although a tendency exists in nursing to choose from among available nursing theories one that is true for us and our practice, to the exclusion of all others, I will not accede to that tendency. Less restrictive and more pertinent to the needs of knowledgeable caring is the alignment and congruence of a number of emerging theoretical frameworks to provide a common ground for nursing practice.

NURSING THEORIES AND THE ENERGETIC BASIS FOR CONSCIOUS CARING

The Rogerian Framework

Martha Rogers' (1970) work lays the foundation. While this work is commonly referred to as nursing theory, it is more truly a worldview that provides a framework from which theories of nursing may be derived. The underlying assumptions of this worldview include: *Man is a unified, irreducible whole.* Human beings are greater than and different from the sum of their parts, and cannot be adequately known, or addressed as systems, organs and cells, as in the medical model. *Man is characterized as a human energy field.* The human energy field encompasses the multiple dimensions of selfhood as an expression of human wholeness. *The unified human energy field is an open system, constantly exchanging matter and energy with the environment. The environment is a greater energy field that extends to infinity.* The whole of each human energy field interacts with the whole of its environment, including other human energy fields, in a dynamic, ongoing energy exchange that is life. We observe and live these exchanges every day—personally and in our nursing practices. Some simple examples of energy exchanges are eating, excreting, speaking, breathing, and emoting. Energy exchanges are simultaneous processes of change and creation unique to each person–environment field; energy exchanges are not cause and effect relationships. *The identity and integrity of the human energy field is maintained through patterning and organization.* The order of life is maintained through constant change. Patterns are seen in rhythmical relationships within each human energy field and between the human and environmental energy fields. We see evidence of this in physiological patterns such as those involved in sleeping–waking, and temperature and hormonal cycles.

Patterns may also be seen in tendencies of thought and spirituality, such as the values, attitudes, and beliefs that are unique to each human energy field. In relation to the environmental field, we see patterns and rhythms of energy exchange such as work, recreation, and family or social alliances.

In this worldview, the concept of homeostasis is obsolete. Rogers' principles of *homeodynamics* add further detail to her framework. According to Malinsky (1986), the principles of homeodynamics "describe the nature and direction of change manifested by unitary human beings in mutual process with the environment" (p. 194). This process is in the direction of greater diversity, complexity, creation, innovation, and fulfillment of potential. Our ability to know ourselves and our world allows us to reflect, choose, and engage consciously in the process of life. As Rogers (1920) states, "The phenomenon central to nursing . . . is the life process in man" (p. 83).

The Rogerian framework, summarized here, describes the universe as energy, and the life process as dynamic energy exchanges on all levels of being. The term *energetics*, as used in this chapter, is based on the Rogerian framework as the context for nursing, and refers to the specific nature of energy exchange that occurs in every act of nursing. As nurses consciously integrate an understanding of the energetics involved in caring for another, they empower the caring role in three ways:

- They minimize the barriers to and hazards of caring.
- They expand their capacity to fulfill the compassionate healer role.
- They potentiate the healing outcomes of those they care for.

The Rogerian Framework Expanded

Other nursing theorists who have built on the Rogerian worldview add detail to the energetics of the caring process and purpose of nursing. Margaret Newman's work, for example, embraces Roger's assumptions and relates them to Bohm's theory of reality as undivided wholeness. According to the physicist Bohm, there is an implicate order, an unseen matrix of energy, underlying reality. Arising from the implicate order is the explicate order, all the tangible phenomena that we know of through our senses. Bohm posits the interplay between the implicate and explicate orders as a process of enfolding and unfolding.

Margaret Newman's Health as Expanding Consciousness

Newman (1989) suggests that the patterns of a person's life include information enfolded from the past, as well as information to unfold in the future. Newman's concept of health as expanding consciousness is a synthesis of the ideas put forward by Roger's and Bohm. Newman identifies consciousness not only as awareness, but also as the overall informational capacity and responsiveness of a human being in the process of enfolding and unfolding within the environment.

Rogers and Newman both define health as a process of manifestation of the rhythmic fluctuations of the life. Health and illness are no longer seen as opposites, one more desirable than the other. Rather, well being and disease are seen as energy fluctuations between order and disorder, organization and disorganization, harmony and disharmony in the life process called health. Likening consciousness to a dissipative structure, Newman (1990) suggests that, at times, we experience giant fluctuations when the old rules no longer seem to work. She envisions nurses as partners to others at these times, supporting clients when asked to choose a medical procedure, that point where transcendence, and learning of new rules, and a higher order of being are most possible.

As nurses assist clients to illumine their patterns, the insight and synchrony the client achieves in the process is healing. Ultimately, it is not our role to control, or to fix anything for another; we bear witness to and engage in the process of expanding consciousness, of both our own and our clients' reality. Our own consciousness becomes a significant factor in the unfolding potentialities.

Rosemarie Parse's Man-Living-Health

Parse (1981) describes this process as Man-Living-Health and identifies aspects of the mutual dance in which the nurse and the client both structure meaning, cocreate patterns, and identify and choose possibilities in the process of enfolding and unfolding, which she terms *cotranscending*. According to Parse, we structure meaning by expressing valued images of reality through language. We come together with and move apart from our clients, connecting and separating, sometimes revealing, sometimes concealing, sometimes enabling, and other times limiting. In Parse's terms, this is the process of transformation which occurs as we "push" some and resist other possibilities in expressing and originating our unique selves in each moment. Parse's work thus adds detail to the energetic framework of conscious caring that is nursing. We can appreciate the complexity of the energetic interplay between nurse and client through her rich languaging of this process.

Jean Watson's Caring-Healing Model

Watson (1988a, b) presents the notion of a transpersonal field of consciousness of the nurse–client, as one field of caring–healing. Watson proposes that transpersonal caring–healing is shared consciousness between a nurse and client, which occurs as an interpenetration of their holographic energies. In effect, there is an interpenetration of the implicate-explicate whole of the nurse, with the implicate-explicate whole of the client, which is inseparable from the implicate-explicate whole of everything. We bring all of who we are to the other when we are in their presence and engage with all of who they are.

Newman (1989) concurs when she so beautifully states, "In the case of a nurse interacting with a patient, the energy fields of the two interact and form a new pattern of inter-penetration, spirit within spirit" (p. 6).

NURSING AND KNOWING

Carper's Ways of Knowing in Conscious Caring

Our awareness of the potential of each encounter is dependent on our consciousness of the implicit and explicit energetics that are transpiring as we engage. In turn, our consciousness is dependent on our facility with the four ways of knowing in nursing that Carper (1978) has described.

Empirical knowing. Empirical knowing of observable, verifiable phenomena is the knowledge of the explicate order, those phenomena that are physically manifest and that may be tangibly experienced and measured. Nurses are typically well trained in the utilization of empirically known factors in their caring activities.

Ethical knowing. For each of us, our personal experience is the frame of reference for the choices we make. Ambiguity, uncertainty, and unpredictability arise as we find ourselves in situations where discernment of right and wrong seem necessary. In nursing we are often involved in another person's process of decision making regarding ethical issues, as well as in the broader matrix of societal energetics around ethical dilemmas. In energy terms, ethical issues and dilemmas may be described as energetic encounters that create ripples as varying points of view collide, or harmonize in their patterns. Conscious awareness of the energetics involved in ethical processes provides perspective which allows nurses to minimize the detrimental forces of ethical collisions, and to facilitate harmonious resolutions.

Esthetic knowing. The perception of abstractions particular to an interaction in the moment, such as the energy dynamics of rhythm, proportion, balance, and unity of a situation, are included in esthetic knowing. Esthetic knowing underlies the art of nursing as it reflects the creative flare of perceiving the whole, aspects of the whole, and the interrelationships there-of. The perceived unity of actions and results, and the personal style which expresses our uniqueness and which we perceive in others, is all encom-passed in esthetic knowing.

Personal knowing.   Self-knowledge, the awareness of self in a given mo-ment, brings one into authentic presence to another as a way of engaging in a relationship. Watson (1990) suggests that true presence reflects an expanded field of consciousness which potentiates one's inner power and resources and, therefore, potentiates healing.

Presence, Caring, and "Not-Knowing"

In the interactions of nurses with clients, a key energetic is presence, a mutual "being with" between nurse and client. True presence often leaves nurses feeling vulnerable and in a state of "not-knowing." Nurses are frequently challenged to energetically stay present and face the unknown and unknow-able with their clients. The discomfort of "not-knowing" raises a need in us to understand transpersonal energetics lest they be perceived as dangerous. Oth-erwise, in order to protect ourselves, we might opt to contract our conscious-ness, limiting the extent to which we are willing to be fully present to the client. This may be understood as self-protection from the energetic occupa-tional hazards of nursing, and may be conscious or unconscious on the part of the nurse.

THE ENERGETIC OCCUPATIONAL HAZARDS OF CARING

This author's background in the study, practice, and teaching of Therapeutic Touch provides a basis for addressing the energetic phenomena involved here. An image presented by Dr. Janet Quinn (1982) in a class she taught on Therapeutic Touch comes to mind. Dr. Quinn said that as nurses walk down the corridor of the hospital, or any setting in which they provide care, they can almost feel the needs of clients reaching out to them, as though the clients are there with fishing rods and reels, casting out as nurses go by and hooking them energetically. "How do nurses deal with this," she asked? An excellent question!

The needs that represent the hooks clients use to snag nurses with are in fact the same reasons nurses are there: to meet the clients' needs which are their call for nursing. Often these needs present as fear and pain, sadness, anguish, loss and grief, or anger, anxiety, and frustration. Of course, nurses also experience, peace, hope, love, surrender, and other poignant moments of human beauty with clients. However, these moments are not as threatening to us as the moments listed initially are.

If we envision the process of being with the client as an energetic engagement, the nature of the threat, the reality of the danger become clear. As nurses openly engage with clients, they experience energetic absorption of their client's fear and pain and resonate with their client's frustration and anger. If the client's need is great, might the client not sap nurses of energy in the client's great need to replenish his or her own. Then, too, there is the potential for nurses to identify with the emotional hurt, spiritual desperation, or depression expressed by clients.

However, these energetics only represent dangers insofar as nurses are unconscious of them, or unprepared to respond in a way that sustains the nurse's capacity to simultaneously nurture the client and the self. The magnitude of this concern grows when we consider the much discussed problems of nursing shortage and burnout in the face of increasing client acuity.

Lack of self-renewal skills and a tendency to empathize with the emotional hurt of clients may lead to a tendency for nurses to energetically withdraw. This may take the form of focusing on tasks and doing, rather than being with, as the primary nursing activity with clients. Additionally, shifting into an objective, authoritative role in which the nurse assumes responsibility and exercises control over clients is another way nurses may attempt to energetically insulate themselves. This is antithetical to the caring role that is the heart of nursing. It undercuts nurses' capacity to be compassionate and surely minimizes the therapeutic value of the nursing interaction for clients.

Gadow (1989) reflects that this is not only something that nurses do in the perceived threatening moments presented here, but is something nurses learn early in their careers. It is easier for nurses to regard clients as objects and take a disembodied view to "avoid embarrassing themselves and the patient, to expedite awkward procedures and to avoid feeling pain when inflicting pain on patients" (p. 537). Gadow observes that nurses learn to regard their own bodies as objects, thereby becoming disembodied caregivers, dissociating from their own bodies in avoidance of experiencing their patient's pain. She further suggests that in order to provide care in the intersubjective framework, nurses must be willing to re-embody, which again raises the issue of vulnerability and safety. Courage and devotion are necessary for nurses to consciously make the choice to be fully present and energetically open in a compassionate way that facilitates wholeness for clients.

Personal and Professional Energy
Management Skills for Nurses

What measures can nurses take to re-embody and stay present? Maintaining conscious awareness of one's own energy field and its dynamics is an excellent beginning. In this regard, Therapeutic Touch offers nurses a mode of clinical intervention as well as personal energy management knowledge and skills. It is possible to identify specific, personalized strategies to protect and renew one's own energy field, using, for example, breathing techniques, self-massage, centering movement, and imagery, all with focused energy oriented intentions.

It is also possible to learn how to channel energy effectively and consciously, to be nurturant on call, so to speak, rather than to distance oneself and maintain detachment out of self-preservation, be it even in the name of caring. It is useful to have a repertoire of self-restoration skills to use if feeling particularly taxed by the energetic fluctuations and disorder we are party to in the lives of others, as well as ourselves.

Nursing education is increasingly including self-study methods for learning centering and presence, use of journaling to explore one's experience of knowing, as well as energy self-support skills, such as those mentioned earlier, in the curricula.

Despite the availability of such methods, the vast majority of practicing nurses are left to their own devices to explore and integrate personal and professional energy management skills. Certainly, studying the current writings of and about the nursing theories presented herein is essential to incorporating them into practice effectively. One way to begin to expand the personal relevance of conscious caring energetics is to retrospectively review one's own lived experience of nursing on a daily basis. At the end of each day look back to at least one nurse–client interaction and ask this question: What was the nature of energy exchanged in that interaction? What was the quality, quantity, and direction of energy exchanged? How did it feel, and what was the outcome, in energetic terms? After a relatively short time of doing this retrospectively, it is common for the nurse to experience this process spontaneously, in the moment, while with clients. The nurse's capacity to engage in conscious caring from an energetic perspective then becomes part of his or her lived experience of nursing, and ongoing self-study.

It is easy to see the vast difference in nature of energy exchange in a common nursing activity, the administration of medication. In the first case, the nurse is preoccupied with personal issues, harried by the demands of the workplace, and unaware of the impact of these pressures on his or her clients as medications are passed impersonally and with haste.

In the second case, the nurse is preoccupied with the same issues, demands, and pressures. However, this nurse chooses to shift his or her consciousness and energy prior to passing through the client's door. The shift is accomplished by breathing deeply, centering, that is, stepping outside of personal issues and consciously focusing on a genuine intention to support the well being of the client while passing medication. No extra time is taken, yet, by bringing conscious awareness of the energetic process into play, this nurse is able to simultaneously extend a more healing, caring presence, and experience the energetic self-renewal of the caring exchange.

SELF-AWARENESS: A KEY FOR CONSCIOUS CARING

Nurses must explore their own consciousness and expand it as a knowledge base for being with clients in their process. We must recognize our own energy patterns and choices in order for clients to reflect on theirs in our presence. Newman (1989) suggests a practice she calls "sensing into one's own field." She states that this involves attending to one's inner experience as a reference for what is occurring in an interaction with a client. In the holographic universe, as we attune more deeply with ourselves, we attune more deeply with the larger context as well.

We must commit to being conscious in the fullness of the transpersonal, holographic energetic interface that is the call for nursing that our clients make. This is necessary not only to maintain our own energetic integrity, but to promote the expansion of consciousness as easily and joyfully as possible for those we serve. This is mastery of the energetics of conscious caring for compassionate healers.

REFERENCES

Carper, B. A. (1978). Fundamental patterns of knowing in nursing. *Advances in Nursing Science*, 13–23.

Gadow, S. (1989). Clinical subjectivity. *Nursing Clinics of North America, 24*, 535–541.

Newman, M. A. (1986). *Health as expanding consciousness*. St. Louis: Mosby.

Newman, M. A. (1989). The spirit of nursing. *Holistic Nursing Practice, 3*(3), 1–6.

Newman, M. A. (1990). Newman's theory of health as praxis. *Nursing Science Quarterly, 3*(1), 37–41.

Parse, R. R. (1981). *Man-Living-Health: A theory of nursing*. Pittsburgh: John Wiley & Sons.

Quinn, J. (1982). *Therapeutic touch: Practice session.* New York: New York University.

Rogers, M. E. (1970). *An introduction to the theoretical basis of nursing.* Philadelphia: F.A. Davis.

Watson, J. (1988a). *Nursing: Human science and human care: A theory of nursing.* New York: National League for Nursing.

Watson, J. (1988b). New dimensions of human caring theory. *Nursing Science Quarterly, 1*(4), 175–181.

Watson, J. (1990). Nursing Theory Conference, Cedars Medical Center, Miami, FL.

6

The Cancer Treatment Experience: Family Patterns of Caring

Patricia J. Larson
Marylin J. Dodd

The experience of cancer treatment places great demands on patients and their families. Initially, issues of cancer diagnosis, treatment decisions, rearrangement of life situations, and strategies for daily maintenance can be challenging to patient and family. If the disease recurs, the family is faced with other challenges that often become major burdens: a changed prognosis, more demanding treatment protocols, and a more acute awareness of the cancer patient's mortality (Cassileth & Hamilton, 1979; Lewis, 1986; Northouse, 1984; Woods, Lewis, & Ellison, 1989). How, then, can family members, facing this emotional burden, rise to the demand of being the mainstay of caring for the person with cancer? It is worthwhile to determine, for example, what a course of chemotherapy requires of a family in caring and what patterns of caring families engage in. With these questions in mind, we reanalyzed a series of interviews we had conducted with family members during cancer patients' chemotherapy.

Caring is defined here as the intentional actions and attitudes that convey physical care, emotional concern, and promote a sense of safeness and security in another. Larsen (1984, 1986, 1987) used this definition of caring, which is focused on patients' practical outcomes, in her inquiries of how nurses convey caring so that patients feel safe and secure.

That the family cares for one of its own when diseased or injured is an implied value. Like the caring associated with nursing, caring within a family is a valued, innate quality that is given spontaneously when a member is faced with a major life challenge. In other words, families, like nurses, will be caring because of the nature of their implied role. However, clinical experiences have taught nurses that appropriate caring does not necessarily occur in families during their experience with cancer.

If caring is conveyed by actions and attitudes, with the intent of promoting a sense of safeness and security in the one cared for, a mutuality of what constitutes caring is implied. In several studies of what constitutes caring, both nurses' and patients' perceptions were examined (Larson, 1987; Mayer, 1987; Keane, Chastain, & Rudisill 1987; von Essen & Sjoden, 1990). The patients consistently ranked the nurse's competency as the most important aspect of caring. The highest rankings were given to the following nurse caring behaviors: getting medications to the patients on time; knowing how to start IVs and how to maintain them; and knowing when to call the doctor. In contrast, nurses consistently ranked as most important: listening, touching, and comforting (Larson, 1984; Mayer, 1987; von Essen & Sjoden, 1990; Keane, Chastain, & Rudisill, 1987). This led us to inquire whether families facing a cancer also hold such divergent views of caring?

Commitment and support to the member diagnosed with cancer takes a toll on families. Studies of families' experience with cancer give evidence that customary roles within the family are often negatively affected (Blank et al., 1989; Quinn & Herndon, 1986; Germino, 1984; Gotay, 1984; Munet, 1984; Vess, Moreland, & Schwebel, 1983; Woods, Lewis, & Ellison, 1985; Wellisch et al., 1978). In addition to family members' worry and concern about the patient's survival, caretaking activities often result in caregiver burden (Hiliman & Lackey, 1990; Haggmark, 1990; Conaster, 1986; Haggmark & Theorell, 1987). Initial treatment experiences affect family interactions and functioning differently than the experience of recurring disease (Gotay, 1984; Woods, Lewis, & Ellison, 1989; Northouse, 1984; Cherkryn, 1984; Krant & Johnson, 1978; Lewis, 1989; Calla, Mahon, & Donovan, 1990; Frank-Stromberg et al., 1984).

Only a few studies report that the experience of cancer has a positive effect on the family. Some spouses became closer, some families became less concerned with materialistic issues, some family members spent more time together (Lieber et al., 1976; Oberst & James, 1985; Northouse & Swain, 1987). These data reveal that husbands and wives were able to share their feelings about the cancer experience. Larger families, however, had greater difficulty communicating about the experience. Evidently, family size and dynamics influence how well they manage the cancer experience.

METHODS

Design

The caring interactions of interest in this study were the actions and attitudes of family members recorded during interviews that focused on problems of or challenges to a family in whom one member received treatment for cancer. Specifically, our analysis addressed: (1) What situations during a family member's course of chemotherapy require the family to demonstrate caring to one another? (2) What the patterns of caring during this experience are? (3) What constitutes meaningful caring for the patient?

A broad definition of family was used in this study so that whomever the patient viewed as family could be included. Thus, the family could be bonded by marriage, birth, or other strong social ties, such as friends and roommates. This broader definition allowed inclusion of the "extended family" common to the West Coast geographical location where the study was conducted.

The data analyzed was generated from interviews with cancer patients and their family members during the patient's course of chemotherapy (Mapes et al., 1990). The interviews were conducted using the Problem-Centered Family Coping Interview (PCFCI) developed by Lewis (1983). The structured PCFCI interview, which is tape recorded and later transcribed verbatim, first has family members share and discuss problems experienced by them during the previous month. These can be on any issue, including but not exclusive to, the chemotherapy experience. The interviewer, who takes field notes to identify which family member generated a problem and who responded and how, guides the family to identify the most important problem. The PCFCI interview format then has the family discuss the effects the problem had on the family, what was done to manage it, and to identify the family members who actively participated in managing the problem. The family is then asked to describe the effects, both positive and negative, the problem or the approach used in solving it had on the family. In reading the data generated from the over 200 PCFCI interviews, Patricia Larson became aware that the data held a wealth of information on whether families did or did not convey caring to one another.

Sample and Setting

The sample consisted of 73 patients, 41 of whom were undergoing initial chemotherapy treatment (24 women and 17 men) and 32 of whom were undergoing chemotherapy for disease recurrence (25 women and 7 men). The majority of women had breast cancer; the men had diagnoses of diverse cancer diseases. Table 6-1 presents the demographic details of the patient sample.

Family units were composed of biological family, spouses, friends, or room-mates. Some families consisted of a dyad, for example, husband and wife, patient and friend, or therapist and lovers. Other family interview groups were comprised of several children, the patient and spouse. Table 6-2 presents the demographics of the families who participated in the interviews.

Table 6-1
Family Demographics: The Patient Sample (N = 73)

	Mean	*SD*	*Range*
Age	48.495	14.147	20–78 years
Education	14.080	2.729	6–20 years

Sex		*Cancer Diagnosis*	
Female	69%	Breast	48%
Male	31%	Lung	10%
Ethnic Background		Colorectal	10%
Asian	7.22%	Gu/Gyn	10%
Black	6.19%	Lymphoma	17%
Caucasian	75.26%	Other	5%
Hispanic	6.19%	Initial cancer treatment	65.26%
Other	3.09%	Recurrence cancer	
Mixed	2.06%	treatment	34.74%
Employment Status			
Full-time*	25.25%	*Marital Status*	
Part-time*	7.07%	Married	58%
Part-time	5.05%	Separated; divorced	17%
Leave of absence	3.03%	Widowed	5%
Disability	14.14%	Single	4%
Not employed	30.30%		
Other	15.15%	*Living Arrangements*	
Primary Family Role		Lives with spouse	50.00%
Mother	43.62%	Lives with other family	
Father	18.09%	members	17.00%
Adult child	6.38%	Lives with significant other	7.00%
Significant other	18.09%	Lives alone	13.00%
Other (roommate, counselor,		Lives with another person	10.00%
etc.)	13.03%	Lives with spouse and family	3.00%

*No change from precancer status

Table 6-2
Family Demographics: The Family Sample (N = 98)

	Mean	SD	Range
Age	42.952	14.732	18–76 years
Education	14.78 yrs	2.991	8–26 years

Sex		*Relationship to Patient (continued)*	
Female	54.76%	Cohabits with significant	
Male	45.24%	other	7.14%
Employment		Neighbor	1.59%
Full-time*	48.00%	Friend	13.49%
Part-time*	12.80%	Other	1.59%
Part-time	2.40%		
Leave of absence	1.60%	*Primary Family Role*	
Disability	3.20%	Mother	21.14%
Not employed other	12.00%	Father	16.26%
Marital Status		Child	14.63%
Married	63.49%	Significant other	22.76%
Separated; divorced	11.90%	Other	22.76%
Widowed	0.79%		
Single	23.81%	*Living Arrangements*	
		Lives with spouse	59.52%
Relationship to Patient		Lives with other family	
Spouse	38.89%	members	12.70%
Child	19.05%	Lives with significant other	11.90%
Sibling	7.14%	Lives alone	9.52%
Parent	6.35%	Other	4.76%
Other relative	4.76%	Lives with spouse and family	1.59%

*No change from before family member's cancer diagnosis

The secondary analysis revealed contextual situations, both family and treatment related, that created the need for caring among family members, and patterns of caring that various family groups used to convey caring to one another. The primary author did the initial interpretation related to the generated caring data, which in turn was examined, clarified, and verified by Marylin Dodd and in consultation with an experienced qualitative researcher. Once consensus was reached, the thematic aspects of each dimension were named.

RESULTS

The data not only generated objective facts about families' problems and management approaches to them, it offered the opportunity to approach the interview data from a secondary analysis perspective using what Wilson (1989) calls "subjective interpretation" (p. 456) whereby the data were allowed to "tell the story," rather than fit a predetermined stance that may influence a critical essence the data holds.

The caring story that emerged from the secondary analysis indicated there are several dimensions to family caring that are associated with a family member's cancer treatment experience. These included family dynamics and patient treatment situations that created a need of "feeling cared for" in one or more family members; the family dynamics and caring approaches used by these families in attempting to meet these needs; and the patterns of family caring that evolved. As noted, family dynamics both created the need for caring as well as influencing how the family (individuals or the family as a whole) attempted to meet or met this caring need. Both positive and negative influences on caring were demonstrated in all these dimensions.

The data reported here reflects the family issues the data revealed. The treatment care demands impacting these families' caring responses are reported elsewhere (Larson & Dodd, 1990).

Family Dynamic and Caring Approaches

The family dynamics that were involved in the caring situations included family make-up (dyad or groups); ages and developmental stages of children and parents; geographical distance between family members; "family-of-choice" or nonbiologically or traditionally bonded family groups; and lifestyle, including job and social situations.

Family make-up was a major contextual issue affecting the giving and receiving of care. Dyadic relations and group interactions appeared to set a different context for family caring to occur. In dyadic relationships, the patient and a significant other often make it easy to convey a sense of mutuality and supportive concern for one another. The dyadic relationship provided the opportunity for direct communication and a simpler approach to problem solving. These dyads often used the term *we*. This "we-ness" conveyed to the patient that there was a partnership in approaching the disease and treatment. The word *we* would often permeate an interview and would be used in referring to treatment decisions, about how lifestyle concerns were dealt with, and discussions of how household chores were managed. The sense of "we-ness" is represented by the following statements: A spouse of a 43-year-old woman with breast cancer said: "We have both discussed it [the diagnosis] and we just kind of help each other out. When I feel sad she tries to help me, and when she is down, then I try to get her up again." The significant other of a 54-year-old lung cancer patient said: "We look at each thing as sort of a hurdle . . . we get over a hurdle and another . . . eventually we'll finish the whole thing together." If present in the first interview, the sense of togetherness would be repeated in the second and third interviews. Togetherness appeared to be a consistently positive force and clearly indicated a mutuality of caring between the two.

Patients whose support came from group interactions of three or more persons were more complex in their caring approach to each other. There were more people and thus more opinions involved in decision making. Consensus on important issues was often difficult to achieve when several family members were involved in the process. Often, there wasn't one particular family member that consistently rallied to the patient's needs. For example, a single 48-year-old man with a diagnosis of throat cancer shared this:

> I'm trying to make my parents understand about my disease but often their mind wanders. My brothers and sisters are concerned but they don't want to talk about the cancer. There is no one in my family that I can open up with or talk to. There are times I really need one of them.

His sister, who participated in the interview, agreed with him, noting that because of her own children's problems she couldn't always be there when her brother needed her.

Young children were often a concern for the cancer parent. The child's need for stability was paramount, but often unfulfilled, such as this 26-year-old lymphoma patient's concern about her 2-year-old:

> My concern is that she's "bouncing." In the daytime she's at someone else's house; at night she's here. She's going between two or three people. Her schedule is all out of whack.

All interviews with families who had school-age or younger children reflected an intense effort to provide consistency for their children, such as regular meals, bed times, and so on. However, the data revealed that this was difficult to maintain and the outcome was often like the above family's dilemma.

Adolescent children, especially those in their late teens or early twenties, wanted to be caring. Their own life demands of college, jobs, and emerging relationships often left a promised commitment undone, such as never getting around to doing their mother's chores on her day of treatment. However, these unfulfilled practical commitments were often tempered by a uniquely touching, caring outreach, such a leaving an "I love you Mom" note in the mother's wig. For this mother, undergoing a rigorous treatment regimen and hating the resulting hair loss, this note made up for all the unfulfilled promises of "help" that were never forthcoming from her daughter. In several instances children away at college would become so overwhelmed with a parent's cancer diagnosis that they began to fall behind in their studies. This then created a situation where they, too, needed caring. Their parent undergoing treatment often was unable to fulfil this need.

The needs of elderly parents were ongoing and often couldn't accommodate to the variations of the adult children's treatment demands. Elderly parents were often not told of progression of the disease of the patient. Women, in particular, whether patient or partner of the patient, tried to maintain ongoing support for elderly parents such as providing meals or transportation. When treatment demands precluded maintaining these activities that had become important or necessary to elderly parents' welfare, a feeling of guilt was often pervasive in the family member who usually provided these services. Often there was no one else to provide this support, so the family member, even if a patient, continued on managing all demands. For many of these patients their need to feel cared for went unfulfilled.

Geographical distance between family members was both a positive and negative force for caring to occur. Because of geographical distance, there was no ongoing family support for some patients who had only intermittent visits from family members. Occasionally, however, geographical distance between family members was perceived as a benefit. Patients with adult children often expressed relief that they did not have to deal with their children's challenging life events on a daily basis. Many of the patients were at the stage in life where their children were beginning to leave home, but were not yet totally independent. Many of these patients kept their adult children informed about events related to their treatment but did not invite them home to "help" during this period. Most patients who did not invite others to come help had a long-standing close-by person, such as a spouse or long-time friend they could regularly count on.

Nonbiological families, often identified in the interviews as "family-of-choice" by a patient whose own family was not wanted or available, were represented in the interviews. Since most "families-of-choice" were comprised of several adults (usually three to four), there was the likelihood that there would always be someone available when the patient needed them. However, their ongoing life commitments often took precedence over their ability or commitment to help care for the patient. This was demonstrated during an interview of a 24-year-old lymphoma patient and her "family-of-choice" roommate. The roommate stated, "I know she needs help on her treatment day, but my wedding plans are at the stage I can't always be there for her." This patient drove herself to and from her treatment, despite the sedation she experienced from the anti-nausea medication she took before and immediately after treatment. In another instance, a patient's best friend who participated in all the interviews, sadly admitted at the third interview that she had not seen her friend (the patient) since the second interview. The patient had been alone for several days after her treatment dealing with a major bout of nausea and vomiting. The friend's work situation did not provide time off for family related matters. Unfortunately, for this patient, this friend was her only family.

Many families spoke to the issue of "maintaining." They had to maintain jobs, lifestyles, and relationships. Treatment demands, as challenging as they were, were often superseded by the need to maintain life commitments. The need to maintain employment for health care insurance, financial security, and desired lifestyle was evident in the great majority of the interviews. For the patients, another reason to remain employed was to demonstrate their value, in spite of having a cancer diagnosis. The following statements convey the dilemmas of maintaining employment. The wife of a 36-year-old patient newly diagnosed with colon cancer said: "My first responsibility is to him. But to do this I need to unscramble my job situation as I have a very high-stress job. I would like to move to a low-stress job, but I'm in conflict, because my present job is only half-time, anything else I can get is full-time and with his situation, it could be quite difficult to change to full-time." A 25-year-old lymphoma patient said: "I'm deciding whether I should keep working. I feel like I can't physically, but mentally I need to keep working. A big part of my identity is my work and I'm afraid to let it go."

Unstable family dynamics such as job loss of a spouse or a close friend, or a crisis for a loved family member was unsettling for all members including the patient. In reality, the patient's treatment experience generally consumed everyone's caring energy. Patients, in particular, needed reassurance that the person in need was receiving help from someone else. Such was the case of a 48-year-old patient whose boyfriend was dealing with an alcohol problem: "My treatments are so upsetting to him. He's started drinking and needs to get back to AA. I just don't have the energy. I so hope our friends will help him." In subsequent interviews it was revealed the man had continued to drink and was finally hospitalized for treatment. Both he and the patient did not experience the desired or needed caring.

Marital and personal relationships also affected the ability to be caring. As noted, stable dyadic relationships were often a positive force in generating caring. However, if there were marital problems prior to the patient's chemotherapy experience, they were rarely resolved during this period, as this husband of a breast cancer patient noted, "Our relationship was having problems before and we've been to a marriage counselor a bunch of times and the issues have nothing to do with breast cancer so when breast cancer came up, it's brought some of these things to a head." Despite this situation, the husband continued to bring his wife for treatment and participated in all three interviews. He apparently bypassed their marital difficulties and conveyed a caring commitment to her. She indicated she was touched by his "hanging-in-there for me."

In contrast, several women began dating while undergoing chemotherapy, and several of the dyad couples were engaged. The data suggested that, depending on the quality and commitment of the relationship, the impact on caring could be positive or negative.

These contextual issues and situations created the need of caring for the patient and family members as well. Each in their own way contributed to the need for the patient to feel cared for. They also, as noted, revealed situations that created a need for caring by other family members such as a husband or child. However, the patient was the one who usually had the greatest need to be cared for. The previously shared statements from patients and their families provide some insight of how this need was manifested, and how individual family members responded to this caring need. Both patient and family members perceived (rightly or wrongly) that because the patient had the cancer and was receiving chemotherapy he or she had the greatest need. The "family-of-choice," in which a dyad or a group of adults were committed to one another, reflected these same patterns of caring.

FAMILY PATTERNS OF CARING

The secondary analysis of this sample of 73 cancer patients and their family members revealed three distinct patterns of caring: sharing, historic and ongoing, and team. The families were quite consistent in maintaining the style of

Sharing
- sense of "we-ness"
- reciprocal caring
- networking

Historic and Ongoing
- established patterns of caring
- being there

Team
- group approach
- mandated caring
- "changing the guard"

Figure 6-1
Family Patterns of Caring

caring they modeled in the first interview during the subsequent two interviews. Figure 6–1 presents the dimension of the families' patterns of caring.

Sharing

Sharing is a mode of family caring that conveys a sense of "we-ness," reciprocation and networking. This sense of "we-ness" as described in the section on dyad's effect on caring was a very positive pattern of family caring. It conveyed to almost everyone, other family members, health care professionals, and so on, that caring was alive and well in the family. During the interviews, both partners conveyed a clear sense that they felt cared for from their mutual interactions.

Reciprocal caring was evident in families who shared the experience of cancer. Patients who knew their constant fatigue was demanding on their partner's time and energy would often talk about saving their own energy reserves to do some special thing for their partner. This exchange about saving energy for pancakes on Saturday is a touching example of how the patient was able to reciprocate her husband's added efforts in helping her through her treatment experience: "What is real important to me is cooking for him. We finally had pancakes last Sunday. The first time in a long time. No sex . . . just pancakes."

The interview data presented several instances of this reciprocal caring by the patient. It was not uncommon to find this reciprocal approach to caring by the several patients who recognized they were terminally ill. A patient, who had stopped her chemotherapy by the third interview because of the extent of her disease, talked about a "book of memories" she was doing for her 4-year-old daughter. "I'm starting a journal telling her what happened between her and me when she was little, even before she was born. Things that nobody knows about but me. I would like her to have those experiences." This woman and others who shared similar caring outreaches conveyed through the interview data that it was very important to be able to complete these endeavors. It was almost as though they wanted to put their sparse energy into caring actions now that they no longer had to fight the cancer.

Although the "we-ness" and reciprocal aspect of caring was most often demonstrated in dyadic relationships, sharing was also present in larger family groups. They too could demonstrate a sense of "we-ness" and reciprocation, although the data demonstrated this happened less often in family groups than in dyads. These families generally showed their caring by establishing a realistic, practical network system to support the patient including conveying the patient's health status, needs, and general happenings to other family and friends. This form of caring appeared to be very important to the patient. The network system, if followed through, provided a buffer for the patient through which selected information could be conveyed, contact times established, and, on several occasions, the orderly procession of when and what food would be welcomed. For a patient with major bouts of nausea and vomiting, unwanted food that was delivered at the wrong time was a major hindrance to feeling safe and secure. Fatigue was another patient symptom that pervaded the interview data. Anything done to decrease the demands on the patient's energy also conveyed a strong sense of caring.

Historic and Ongoing

Historic and ongoing care was generally represented by interactions among larger family groups; these occurred between parents and adult children. Several families clearly had experienced and conveyed caring throughout the years and in many situations. They represented, in a sense, "experienced caring." They knew what things were meaningful to one another, and they knew when to back off. They often declared "we're a caring family, you know," and then would go on to tell some anecdote: "We are a close family. Today they were all here and we know each other well. When anything happens we call each other. We always help one another." They seemed to have established a rhythm to easily convey caring to one another. Who needed to be cared for was readily perceived and the needed caring action or attitude enacted.

The sense of having a historic and ongoing commitment was not restricted to family units with relationships established over a long period of time. Young couples who had only been together for a short period, or a friendship that had recently evolved would convey this supportive mode of caring. For example, two women who had recently met through a running club participated in the interviews as a family. The nonpatient stated: "I want to be there for her, it's important to me. I'm certain that if it were me, she'd do the same for me."

Perhaps the basic premise of the families' sharing or historic and ongoing commitments to one another was that they would be there for one another. One almost could gain a sense of calmness and security from the patients who had this kind of family backup. Both forms of caring, sharing and historic and ongoing, were quite effective in making the patient feel cared for. What mode of caring was more effective did not become clear from the interviews. However, it was made clear that these caring models were more effective in conveying caring than the team model or third pattern of family caring that evolved from the data.

Team Caring

Team caring conveyed a dynamic family force that, as it seemed, mandated "caring" to the patient. However, this sort of caring often overwhelmed the patient. For example, if the patient was the parent, and the team caring was generated by their energetic, well-meaning, but disorganized children, the parent patient often needed to calm or defuse volatile situations at a time when he or she had little energy to do so. This was demonstrated by a family scenario, described in interview, in which a woman, newly treated for breast cancer, had her three adult children quit their jobs and come home to be with her. Three interviews, reflecting a six-month period in their life, revealed that these well-meaning children were often unable to find jobs. When they did work they often had conflicting hours and only one car to share. Over the course of time, money became ever more of a problem. The mother's treatment and management of side effects became points of conflict. Throughout the interviews, however, the participating children would frequently state that they were "a caring family." The mother did not participate in the interviews unless prompted to by one of the research assistants, only to be interrupted when she did speak by one of her children. Although everyone involved in her care seemed well intentioned, the question remains. Did adequate caring occur?

"Changing the guard," another form of team caring, was also problematic for patients in achieving a sense of safeness and security. Changing the guard is best demonstrated by a plan for helping a young woman with lymphoma that was shared by her boyfriend: "I am usually here but when I had to study for finals I often needed to go to the library, so her mom came. That worked out pretty well. Then her mom had to get back to her job and her father and his wife came. They treated her [patient] like a little child. The resulting conflict got pretty tough." Although all these people were important to the patient it was obviously disconcerting for her to have to deal with so many different people and attitudes. However, in today's reality of obligations to jobs and other commitments, "changing the guard" may continue to be a reality. As problematic as "changing the guard" was for the families involved, the fact that family members were interested in and willing to help was often quite touching to patients. They seemed to feel both cared for and overwhelmed.

The sharing, historic, and ongoing patterns of caring represented positive processes utilized by families in dealing with problems they encountered during a course of a family member's chemotherapy. Family members were usually effective in solving problems and conveying caring to one another. Team caring was somewhat less effective, both in achieving problem solving and conveying caring. However, there were several instances where caring was needed, when an individual desperately needed to feel cared for but the caring never was demonstrated. Here the interview data revealed several challenges to caring.

Challenges to Caring

Secondary analysis revealed family dynamics that were major challenges to caring. Figure 6-2 presents the critical challenges to caring among family members, including instances where there really wasn't a family unit, only an "imagined" family, or when there were long-standing chaotic relationships among family members. When unexpected disease progression occurred, there were several family members who could not rally caring effectively for the patient. This effect is describe elsewhere (Larson & Dodd, 1990).

Issues of family dynamics that almost precluded any hope that the patient would feel cared for did arise. For example, to participate in the study, patients had to designate someone as family. Some single persons selected long-term friends for their family unit. But several patients selected casual friends or roommates as "family." These casual or "imagined" family members rarely conveyed an ongoing caring commitment to the patient. Although they indicated they recognized the patient's plight, they were also quite clear in saying that they were there for an interview, or for a specific situation, rather than committing themselves further. As a result, those patients who named casual or imagined family members as caregivers were essentially on their own.

Strained relationships, especially in those families with an extensive conflictive history, generally did not work to rally a caring response when one of their members received a diagnosis of cancer. This quote from a 35-year-old patient with recurrence of breast cancer is typical here: "My mother doesn't speak to me at the moment. She just can't cope with my situation. I can't get out of bed in the morning and yet she wants me to come down and help her."

- "imagined" family
- long-standing relationships
- strained relationships

Figure 6-2
Challenges to Caring Among Family Members

DISCUSSION

The limitations of secondary analysis of qualitative data must be acknowledged. Although the data provided a unique opportunity for analysis of families' accounts of their experiences of dealing with the impact of disease and treatment, and thus were valuable in suggesting areas that merit further study, there was no opportunity for exploration of emerging hypotheses with patients and their selected family members or theoretical sampling to saturate categories, or for respondent validation of our conclusions. Since these procedures are regarded as important for checking on the validity of the analysis, the findings described above are presented with the caveat that they are suggestive only. Additional data collection is necessary to warrant more definitive conclusions. Nevertheless, and despite these limitations, the PCFCI family interviews provided valuable insight into how family members demonstrate caring to one another. Further research will determine if these interpretations of family caring hold true.

One further note need be mentioned here. The PCFCI interviews revealed very little positive or negative nursing influence on these families. This may be because the interviews focused only on the family. However, the data were rich with stories, albeit negative at times, about the impact physicians and the health care setting and system had on the patients' and families' experiences. Nursing's role was alarmingly silent. Further research is needed to corroborate this finding.

As noted, the limitations of this secondary analysis preclude any major generalization to nursing practice. They do, however, provide a message that practitioners should heed. First, the family of the cancer patient is important. Most families want to be involved and are needed for their support to the patient. The data from this study, like other studies on families of patients with cancer, show that families also have needs of their own.

Family members should be informed and guided on realistic approaches to the patient. Data from this study indicates that it may be particularly important to identify the key family member who will be the main support of the patient for a course of treatment. This person will need special sensitivity and support from health care providers so that he or she will not be unduly burdened. Larger family units may need assistance in developing realistic approaches to processing their caring endeavors. For example, a family conference with all interested family members and the patient could be held where the patient's treatment plan would be outlined, including projected times when the patient will need assistance in getting to treatment and the managing of treatment side effects, such as nausea and vomiting or fatigue. Family members could then begin to plan practical approaches in assisting the patient. With the entire family together, and with supportive guidance from the nurse, they could develop strategies realistic to their lifestyle, and still provide adequate caring support for the patient. It would be interesting, of course, to see if such strategies would also temper the burden that many cancer families experience during a family member's experience of cancer.

For those interested in caring, and committed to the concept that all patients need to feel cared for, it is essential that research on caring be continued. This study provides evidence that caring within family groups occurs as it indicates that for some patients their needed caring cannot be met by their real or imagined family. Clinical methods must be explored to help these persons. Existing help, at least in terms of transportation as provided by the American Cancer Society, may be a realistic initial resource. In addition, the volunteer services of health care organizations could find treatment partners for cancer patients, in programs somewhat akin to hospice volunteers. Patients undergoing treatment need and deserve to feel cared for. The experience of cancer treatment is truly too challenging to be faced alone.

REFERENCES

Blank, J. J., Clark, L., Longman, A. J., & Atwood, J. R. (1989). Perceived home care needs of cancer patients and their caregivers. *Cancer Nursing, 12*(2), 78–84.

Cassileth, B. R., & Hamilton, J. N. (1979). The family with cancer. In B. R. Cassileth (Ed.), *The cancer patient: social and medical aspects of care.* (pp. 233–247). Philadelphia: Lea & Febiger.

Cella, D. F., Mahon, S. M., & Donovan, M. I. (1990). Cancer recurrence as a traumatic event. *Behavioral Medicine,* 15–22.

Chekryn, J. (1984, December). Cancer recurrence: Personal meaning, communication, and marital adjustment. *Career Nursing.*

Conatser, C. (1986). Preparing the family for their responsibilities during treatment. *Cancer, 58,* 508–511.

Degner, L. F., & Aquino-Russell, C. (1988). Preferences for treatment control among adults with cancer. *Research in Nursing & Health, 11,* 367–374.

Drew, N. (1986). Exclusion and confirmation: A phenomenology of patients' experiences with caregivers. *Image: Journal of Nursing Scholarship, 18*(2), 39–43.

Frank-Stromberg, M., Wright, P., Segalla, M., & Diekman, J. (1984). Psychosocial impact of the "cancer diagnosis." *Oncology Nursing Forum, 11*(3), 16–22.

Germino, B. (1984). *Family members' concerns after cancer diagnosis.* Doctoral Dissertation. University of Washington, Seattle.

Knafl, K. A., & Deatrick, J. A. (1986). How families manage chronic conditions: An analysis of the concept of normalization. *Research in Nursing & Health, 9*, 215-222.

Krant, M., & Johnston, L. (1978). Family members' perception of communications in late stage cancer. *International Journal of Psychiatry in Medicine, 8*(2), 203-216.

Larson, P. L. (1984). Cancer Patients' Perceptions of Important Nurse Caring Behaviors. *Oncology Nursing Forum, 11*(6), 46-50.

Larson, P. L. (1986). Cancer Nurses' Perceptions of Caring. *Cancer Nursing, 9*(2), 86-91.

Larson, P. L. (1987). Comparison of Cancer Patients' and Professional Nurses' Perceptions of Important Nurse Caring Behaviors. *Heart and Lung, 16*(2), 187-193.

Larson, P., & Dodd, D. (1990). Cancer treatment demands on family caring. (In review).

Lewis, F. M. (1983). *Problem centered family coping interviews.* Seattle: University of Washington.

Lewis, F. (1986). The impact. *Patient Education and Counseling, 8*(3), 269-289.

Lewis, F. M. (1989). Attributions of control, experienced meaning, and psychosocial well-being in patients with advanced cancer. *Journal of Psychosocial Oncology, 7*(1/2), 105-118.

Lieber, L., Plumb, M. M., Gertenzang, M. L., & Holland, J. (1976). The communication of affection between cancer patients and their spouses. *Psychosomatic Medicine, 38*, 379-389.

Loescher, L. J., Welch-McCaffrey, D., Leigh, S. A., Hoffman, B., & Meyskens, F. L. (1989). Surviving adult cancers. Part I: Physiologic effects. *Annals of Internal Medicine, 111*, 411-432.

Loescher, L. J., Welch-McCaffrey, D., Leigh, S. A., Hoffman, B., & Meyskens, F. L. (1989). Surviving adult cancers. Part II: Psychosocial implications. *Annals of Internal Medicine, 111*, 517-524.

Mapes, D., Price, M., Kesselring, A., & Dodd, M. (1990). Critique of a family interview technique. *Proceedings of the 23rd Annual Communicating Nursing Research Conference, Western Society for Research In Nursing,* Denver, Colorado.

Mayer, D. K. (1987). Oncology nurses' versus cancer patients' perceptions of nurse caring behaviors: A replication study. *Oncology Nursing Forum, 14*(3), 48-51.

Munet de Vilaro, F. (1984). *Coping strategies and adaptation to childhood cancer of Puerto Rican families.* Doctoral Dissertation. University of Washington, Seattle.

Northouse, L. L. (1981). Mastectomy patients and the fear of recurrence. *Cancer Nursing, 4*(3), 213-219.

Northouse, L. (1984). The impact of cancer on the family: An overview. *International Journal of Psychiatry in Medicine, 14*(3), 215-242.

Northouse, L. (1984). The impact of cancer on the family: An overview. *International Journal of Psychiatry in Medicine, 14*(3), 215-242.

Northouse, L. L., & Swain, M. A. (1987). Adjustment of patients and husbands to the initial impact of breast cancer. *Nursing Research, 36*, 221-225.

Northouse, L. L. (1989). The impact of breast cancer on patients and husbands. *Cancer Nursing, 12*(5), 276-284.

Oberst, M., & James R. (1985). Going home: Patient and spouse adjustment following cancer. *Topics in Clinical Nursing, 7,* 46-57.

Olesen, V. L. (1989). Caregiving, ethical and informal: Emerging challenges in the sociology of health and illness. *Journal of Health and Social Behavior, 30,* 1-10.

Peterson, B. H. (1985). A qualitative clinical account and analysis of a care situation. In M. M. Leininger (Ed.), *Qualitative research methods in nursing,* (pp. 267-281). New York: Grune & Stratton.

Quinn, W. H., & Herndon, A. (1986). The family ecology of cancer. *Journal of Psychosocial Oncology, 4*(1/2), 45-59.

Stetz, K. M., Lewis, F. M., & Primono, J. (1986). Family coping strategies and chronic illness in the mother. *Family Relations, 35,* 515-522.

Theorell, T., Haggmark, C., & Eneroth, P. (1987). Psycho-endocrinological reactions in female relatives of cancer patients. Effects of an activation programme. *Acta Oncol, 26,* 419-424.

Thorne, S. (1985). The family cancer experience. *Cancer Nursing, 8*(5), 285-291.

Vess Jr., J. D., Moreland, J. R., & Schwebel, A. I. (1985). An empirical assessment of the effects of cancer on family role functioning. *Journal of Psychosocial Oncology, 3*(1).

von Essen, R., & Sjoden, P. (1990). Nurses' versus patients' perceptions of nurse caring behaviors: A replication study. *Centre for Caring Sciences.* Uppsala, Sweden: Akademiskasjukhuset.

Weisman, A. D., & Worden, J. W. (1976). The existential plight in cancer: Significance of the first 100 days. *International Journal of Psychiatry in Medicine, 7*(1), 1-15.

Wellisch, D. K., Fzwzy, F. I., Landsverk, J., Pasnau, R. O., & Wolcott, D. L. (1983b). Evaluation of psychosocial problems of the homebound cancer patient: The relationship of disease and the sociodemographic variables of patients to family problems. *Journal of Psychosocial Oncology, 1*(3), 1-15.

Wilson, H. S. (1989). Research in Nursing. Redding, MA: Addison-Wesley.

Woods, N. F., Lewis, F. M., & Ellison, E. S. (1989). Living with cancer. *Cancer Nursing, 12*(1), 28-33.

Woods, N. F., Yates, B. C., & Primono, J. (1989). Supporting families during chronic illness. *Image: Journal of Nursing Scholarship, 21*(1), 46-50.

Worden, J. W. (1989). The experience of recurrent cancer. *CA-A Cancer Journal for Clinicians, 39*(5), 305-310.

7

Expressions of Nurses' Caring: The Role of the Compassionate Healer

Gwen Sherwood

It was a couple of nights ago I really got distended. I had excruciating pain, so much that I was crying out and I was able to get the nurse on the buzzer. She came in and she could see that my belly was as big as a basketball and I was gasping for breath and having a lot of distress. She didn't make any comment. She turned on her heels and went out the door and it wasn't two minutes she was back with, I guess, four doctors, three males and a female. They gave a good examination, decided I didn't need a Levine tube, but gave instructions to the nurse what to do and even though she had the man in the bed next to me, and he's in bad shape, she spent time with me until she made me as comfortable as possible and that was a real neat experience. I knew that I was hurting bad and she was there with me until I felt better. I didn't feel better for some hours, but I had the feeling, that concern when they know what's going on and they are taking care of me and, contrary to public opinion, I'm not going to die.

A patient's world can be a frightening place. Because it is often up to the nurse to instill the gift of hope, the calmness of reassurance, and the promise of recovery, the nurse–patient interaction is most crucial. Nonetheless, while the role of the nurse as the caring, compassionate healer is vital to patient well being, and has been frequently written about, its systematic study is limited.

Since the 1800s when Florence Nightingale wrote of the art of nursing, caring has been a dominant feature in the language of nursing. The nurse-patient interaction comprised of elements both verbal and nonverbal, the repertoire of skilled procedures, and the reassuring touch remains the essential, and potentially most rewarding, aspect of nursing.

Yet the expression of caring in nursing faces increasing challenges. The expanding applications of technology compounded by the demands of the nursing shortage have created a climate which submerges the caring ethic. In today's marketplace as well, *rewards* and *incentives* involve cost-effective treatment modalities and efficient use of time and personnel. But where, as Leininger (1986) has pointed out, is the line item in the budget for caring?

In the effort to advance findings by other nurse researchers (Henry, 1975; Brown, 1986; Larson, 1987; and Riemen, 1986) who have investigated caring from patient perspectives, this study was designed to discover patient descriptions of nurses' caring. Unlike previously reported work, the design allowed for open-ended interviews from hospitalized patients to form the data set. In this way, we can uncover, without researcher or questionnaire suggestion, the essentials of nurses' caring.

PERSPECTIVES ON CARING

Examination of literature from social scientists and philosophers establishes caring in varied perspectives. As existential knowing, Fromm (1956) interprets caring interactions as helping the recipient to overcome separateness and achieve union. Here, caring is understood as an art requiring the deepest knowledge of the person and incorporating effort, respect, and responsibility.

Caring also involves growth enhancement. Mayerhoff (1971) interprets caring as helping people grow. Here, caring is understood as a measure of personhood, which occurs only when the recipient of care is recognized and experienced as a person. One must know the person to understand the other's needs and transform that knowledge into action.

The French philosopher Gabriel Marcel (1981) interprets caring as more than physical presence. Here, existential presence involves availability, openness, and a giving to the other so that a sense of value and respect are communicated.

These perspectives, which form the basis for the concept of caring, highlight the need for the study of caring in nursing. Specialization and the impact of science and technology have made human-to-human interaction an issue to which nurses must pay close attention for the preservation of human caring. Nursing is challenged to reaffirm the human scope of caring as an essential concept in nursing. Research efforts are necessary for explication of the operational parameters of this important concept.

DESIGN OF THE STUDY

To enlarge the scope of knowledge about caring in nursing, a phenomenological study to investigate caring from the perspective of the patient was undertaken (Sherwood, 1988). The study purported to identify and describe patient perceptions of demonstrations of nurses' caring through phenomenological analysis as set forth by Spiegelberg (1976). The convenience sample was comprised of ten post-operative adult patients, five male and five female, selected to reveal a population of patients requiring significant numbers of nursing interactions.

Phenomenology, the qualitative research method for the study of lived experience, allows researcher interviews of participants using open-ended questions. Later analysis of interviews yields patterns developed into themes describing nurses' caring. Here, data analysis involves a simultaneous process of intuiting, analyzing, and describing while the researcher brackets previous knowledge of the phenomenon from conscious thought. Briefly summarized, the steps in data analysis include reading and rereading the transcripts to capture the essence of the interviews. Descriptive words and phrases are highlighted and studied for identification of common themes describing the phenomenon. As themes are identified, descriptive elements are enumerated, adding clarity and meaning to fully show the essence of the phenomenon under study.

INTERPRETATION OF FINDINGS

Analysis of the data yielded responses to the major question of the study: "What do patients perceive as demonstrations of nurses' caring?" Five themes emerged as essential to a demonstration of nurses' caring, each given further meaning and clarification through descriptive elements, including: assessing needs, planning care, intervening, validating, and interacting. While listed sequentially, it must be noted the themes were dynamic and fluid, with movement back and forth, but always present.

Theme 1: Assessing needs was described as assessing what was needed by the patient and was accomplished through three descriptive elements. As observation, the nurse checked frequently for signs and symptoms of distress, pain, discomfort, or other needs. Knowing the nurse was available for observing and assessing gave the patient assurance of assessment. The nurse must give existential presence—be present in mind as well as in body—to sharpen the focus and attention necessary for in-depth knowing of the patient for accurate assessment. As was stated by one participant, "I need to know they are interested in me and are checking on me."

Theme 2: Planning care was summarized as using the nurse's formal preparation and scientific knowledge to establish a plan for managing the patient's care. Scientific knowledge formed the basis of the plan of care with the nurse able to make sound decisions based on observations and information from the assessment. Judgments were based on scientific knowledge of appropriate treatment modalities resulting in knowledgeable decision making in forming the plan of care. The participants expressed a feeling of the nurse being in charge of the overall plan of care, skillfully guiding what was happening, exemplified by the statement, "They are prepared."

Theme 3: Intervening was the implementation of the plan of care by the nurse with appropriate choice of intervention. Assessment, need identification, and a plan of care were not sufficient. For caring to have occurred, the nurse must act on his or her knowledge of the patient's needs and do something to alleviate the problem or need.

Participants considered the nurse's ability to perform skilled nursing procedures a necessary element of nurses' caring. Participants expected the nurse to perform the skill quickly, painlessly, and competently, choosing the appropriate procedures to resolve a need.

Participants viewed the routine things done by the nurse as demonstrations of caring, including checking vital signs, helping with the bath, changing the bed, encouraging activity, serving meals, keeping side rails up, enabling sleep, giving medications on schedule, and, as one patient stated, "Just doing their regular routine." A caring nurse encouraged activity and movement as a means of recuperation and encouraged a return to self-care which was seen as leading toward recovery. Offering help and assistance when needed was a vital communication of caring.

Assistance with mental and physical comfort was a primary concern to participants as well. Descriptions included assisting with pain relief, prevention of nausea, smooth sheets, cleanliness, a comfortable environment, and comfortable body alignment.

Participants valued personalized attention. Talking in a personalized, comforting manner, listening actively to what the patient said, and responding appropriately communicated caring. It was important to offer reassurance of condition, of the nurse's availability, and of the efforts on behalf of the patient. Touch communicated comfort, kindness, and love, and aided alertness. The nurse provided information through patient education and teaching; the nurse's offering explanations to both patient and family was important.

When the nurse did something above and beyond the usual routine, it was considered extra effort and a demonstration of personalized care. Included were such actions as contacting the physician, helping with a personal problem, helping family members, getting needed personal items, protecting modesty, taking care of little things, doing comfort measures, and showing personal interest. As one participant stated:

> I've been in the last 24 hours on a liquid diet. When last evening came I felt great. This morning came, I felt better. A nurse came in and I told her that I got my liquid meal, but I'm hungry. She said, "Let me see if I can do something about that." Within five minutes, Dr. X was in the room and he said, "If you're feeling that good, let's order you a general diet." The nurse could have waited for the doctor to come in, but she took it on herself to find the doctor and tell him, "xxx's done away with his liquid meal, but he wants some solid food." She didn't have to do this because he would have made his rounds in an hour or two. I call that "caring." Being hospitalized in the past in other places, I don't know if people had gone that far.

Theme 4: Validating, evaluating if needs were met, was the fourth theme in a demonstration of caring. The nurse must have followed through with additional care or a revised plan when needs were not met. Patients told of the nurse returning on many occasions to validate the effectiveness of nursing interventions and to check on the patient's condition. "They came back to check on me" was a comment heard frequently. Information elicited provided the basis for revision of the care plan or for further action by the nurse in continuing to seek resolution of the problem or need.

Theme 5: Interacting with the patient with a particular attitude was an essential overall theme. To demonstrate caring, the nurse's actions must be done with certain interactional attitudes having connotations of concern, empathy, kindness, comfort, and personal regard. Without these particular attitudes in the nurse's approach to the patient, the nurse's actions became mere technical expressions, lacking that ingredient necessary for the nurse to demonstrate caring.

Nurse caring, then, is more than just nursing *care*, the *doing* of care for patients. When the appropriate attitude of interaction is a part of nursing care, it becomes nurse caring in all of its dimensions. In giving further meaning to this theme, descriptive elements included concern for comfort and well being, respect and compassion for the individual as a whole person, having regard for feelings, and paying attention to "little things."

Caring nurses acted and spoke with an attitude of kindness and compassion, treating patients gently. Tone of voice did have an impact on patients. It was important for nurses to give their names as well as to call the patient by name. Patients cited expressions of empathy as measures of how well the nurse understood their experience. Personalization of nursing care was demonstrated by having a patient-centered orientation, treating the patient on a person-to-person basis, showing interest in the patient's family, and calling the patient by name.

Participants noted that demonstrations of commitment to professional ideals gave evidence of a nurse's sincere effort to offer the best care possible. Patience—the spending of time necessary to meet the need without rushing—also was important. Another important aspect to caring that arose was a connotation of mothering in a context of the protective, loving aspect of caring.

Participants in the study spoke of caring as the actions and interventions of the nurse performed with an overall positive attitude assistive to the patient. A patient gave this testimony of a positive attitude that aided recovery.

> And then when this one, this one's really good, the one that's on duty right now. She came in, right away I just felt that my feelings mattered and she just was friendly to me in her voice, and her voice is very gentle and soothing and I felt immediately better, just by knowing that she was here. It makes a world of difference, especially if you don't have family, cause we're from out of town, so it's just my husband and myself, so we look for comfort from anyone. It comes from the nurses.

As shown by this study, caring can be described and identified when these five themes encompass what the nurse does. Nurses demonstrate caring when they express an overall attitude of concern, compassion, and commitment through their actions. Knowledgeable assessment of patient needs is, of course, the necessary first step. The plan of care is then personalized with appropriate choice of interventions which lead the client toward a sense of positive well being. In a situation when patient needs are not met, action outcomes are evaluated with validation of patient response so that alternative actions can be implemented.

RELATIONSHIP TO OTHER NURSING PERSPECTIVES ON CARING

The findings of this study are consistent with Koldjeski's (1990) determination of interconnections of professional caring as the identified holistic indicators are unified into a whole: Being (presence, experiencing, actualizing, expressing, compassion, concern, love); Relating (personally, interpersonally, transpersonally); and Doing (professional nursing decisions and actions— nursing therapeutics). These are expressed through a special kind of relation involving being, relating, and doing.

The nurse then functions in a dual aspect of being and doing, of combining scientific knowledge and compassion, action combined with healing. To further understand the nurses' caring within the role of the compassionate healer, these findings were then related to other published work.

Appleton (1990) writes that human care as a way of being concerned suggests that an attitude of compassion is necessary for conveying the caring expression. Thus, caring expressions are a way of being concerned for self and others through expressions arising from a compassionate attitude. According to Appleton, caring involves four themes consistent with the themes found in this study: Treating, Understanding, Helping, and Letting, all surrounded by Compassionate Being, showing both intent and action, being and doing.

The description of nurse caring given here fits with the philosophical analysis of caring as developed by Gaut (1983), who suggests that, in caring, there is an action component and an intention. While the action includes setting goals, choosing tactics to meet goals, and implementing these tactics with skill, the action also must be done with the intention of producing positive changes in the patient.

Watson (1985) speaks of human caring as originating in an attitude which must become something more: a will, an intention, a commitment, and a conscious judgment that manifests itself in concrete acts. A moral intention and the value placed on human life by the nurse will produce positive changes in the patient.

Roach (1984) describes the attitudes of caring as the five Cs. Caring is expressed in *compassionate* and *competent* acts, in relationships qualified by *confidence*, through an informed, sensitive *conscience*, and through *commitment* and fidelity. Again, these broad categories encompass the intent and action, the being and doing aspect of nursing, the defined role of the compassionate healer.

These attributes reflect the role of compassion in healing where one human being responds to another. Prior (1990) views compassion as a motivator, with the caregiver being moved to action. Good intentions are not sufficient but must be coupled with the appropriate actions, determined by one's knowledge and applied through one's skill. Seeing the plight of the individual but not taking appropriate action is not caring. The compassionate healer assesses, plans, intervenes, validates, and interacts for the positive good of the patient.

CONCLUSION

As addressed by Norris (1990), the moral ideal of nursing just described raises one serious question not to be overlooked. Norris asks: Can 1.5 million nurses deliver care or be caring on a regular basis in their relationships with 26 million patients per year? While it is unrealistic to think we will be able to achieve this high standard with all patients, that should not discourage us from pursuing our ideal role of compassionate healer.

As professional nurses, it is our responsibility to model for ourselves and others *how* to care in an increasingly impersonal, technological, and violent world often devoid of compassion and caring. We must begin from a nursing management and administration perspective which values and rewards caring values in nursing (Ray, 1987). We will not have nurturing and caring at the bedside if we fail to nurture and care for ourselves and our colleagues. As compassionate healers, our call to consciousness is to develop systems of nursing delivery consistent with our philosophy of caring, to model for our students a caring mode of being, and to emphasize that skill and knowledge are only parts of the caring model. Social values and bureaucratic structures do make caring difficult when efficiency and cost reductions are the prevailing reward incentives.

Spencer Michael Free's poem illustrates the transitory nature of the outside world, demonstrating the lasting impression of the existential human touch which transcends the physical. The being mode of the compassionate healer is a critical ingredient of caring demonstrations in nursing.

The Human Touch

'Tis the human touch in this world that counts,
The touch of your hand and mine,
Which means far more to the fainting heart
Than shelter and bread and wine;
For shelter is gone when the night is o'er
and Bread lasts only a day,
But the touch of the hand and the sound of the voice
sing on in the soul alway.

Spencer Michael Free

REFERENCES

Appleton, C. (1990). The meaning of human care and the experience of caring in a university school of nursing (77–94). In M. M. Leininger & J. Watson (Eds.), *The caring imperative in education* (pp. 45–58). New York: National League for Nursing.

Brown, L. (1986). The experience of care: Patient perspectives. *Topics in Clinical Nursing, 8*(2), 56–62.

Free, S. M. (1936). The human touch. In H. Felleman (Ed.), *The best loved poems of the American people* (p. 130). Garden City, NY: Doubleday.

Fromm, E. (1956). *The art of loving*. New York: Harper & Row.

Gaut, D. A. (1983). Development of a theoretically adequate description of caring. *Western Journal of Nursing Research, 5*, 313–324.

Henry, O. M. (1975). Nurse behaviors perceived by patients as indicators of caring. *Dissertation Abstracts International, 1976*, 34-B.

Koldjeski, D. (1990). Toward a theory of professional nursing caring: A unifying perspective. In M. M. Leininger & J. Watson (Eds.), *The caring imperative in education* (pp. 45–58). New York: National League for Nursing.

Larson, P. J. (1987). Comparison of cancer patients' and professional nurses' perceptions of important nurse caring behaviors. *Heart and Lung, 16*, 187–193.

Leininger, M. M. (1986). Care facilitation and resistance factors in the culture of nursing. *Topics in Clinical Nursing, 8*(2), 1–12.

Marcel, G. (1981). *The philosophy of existence* (R. Grabon, Ed. & Trans.). Philadelphia: University of Pennsylvania Press.

Mayerhoff, M. (1971). *On caring*. New York: Harper & Row.

Norris, C. (1989). To care or not to care—Questions! Questions! *Nursing and Health Care, 10*(10), 544–550.

Prior, W. (1990). Compassion: A critique of moral rationalism. In R. Taylor & J. Watson (Eds.), *They shall not hurt* (pp. 33–52). Boulder, CO: Colorado Associated University Press.

Ray, M. S. (1987). Health care economics and human caring in nursing: Why the moral conflict must be resolved. *Family and Community Health, 10,* 35–43.

Riemen, D. J. (1986). The essential structure of a caring interaction: Doing phenomenology. In P. L. Munhall & C. J. Oiler (Eds.), *Nursing research: A qualitative perspective* (pp. 85–108). Norwalk, CT: Appleton-Century-Crofts.

Roach, Sr. M. S. (1984). *Caring: The human mode of being, implications for nursing.* Toronto: University of Toronto.

Sherwood, G. (1988). Nurses' caring as perceived by post-operative patients: A phenomenological study. *Dissertation Abstracts International, 49*(06), 2133. (University Microfilms No. ADG88-16567)

Spiegelberg, H. (1976). *The phenomenological movement.* The Hague: Martinus Nijhoff.

Watson, J. (1985). *Nursing: Human science and human care, a theory of nursing.* Norwalk, CT: Appleton-Century-Crofts.

8

Caring and the Story: The Compelling Nature of What Must Be Told and Understood in the Human Dimension of Suffering

Carol Picard

Caring is relational. It is attending to a person's wholeness. Martin Buber (1958) describes the I-Thou relationship as a mutual relation that binds one to the wholeness of other. I-It relationships are the world of experience, not relation, the world of other as object. Sister Simone Roach (1987) defines caring as "the human mode of being" (p. 133). She identifies compassion as the first of her five caring attributes. Her definition of compassion is "a way of living . . . engendering a response of participation in the experience of another" (p. 58).

Jean Watson (1988) describes transpersonal caring as that in which we can enter the experience of another and they into our experience. Appreciating time—past, present, and future of participants in the caring encounter—is vital to her theory.

Cassell (1982) has written on the nature of suffering and the need to attend to the patient's subjective experience, to extend to the patient care with compassion. To attempt to objectify and categorize this experience only diminishes what we can learn from patients. To be a caring, compassionate healer, to enter an I-Thou relationship, we must appreciate *story*.

THE STORY

What is story? Story is an ongoing narrative of events—a history—that includes the meanings a particular person gives to lived events. In Sally Gadow's (1990) words, story includes a person's interior and exterior landscape. It is as particular as theory is generalized. It is our biography as we understand it. According to Benner and Wrubel (1989), care is perceived by patients to include our deep understanding of them based on knowledge derived from our professional education and our clinical practice, as well as from hearing their story.

Norman Cousins (1989), in his book, *Head First: The Biology of Hope*, describes a survey of people living in the University of California at Los Angeles (UCLA) Medical Center area. He found 85 percent of 1,050 persons in the survey had changed physicians over the past five years or were about to change physicians. Why? His data can be summed up in the idea that the patient's story is not being heard. The I-Thou relationship was missing. The respondents made it clear that diagnostic and treatment competence were not at issue.

UNDERSTANDING ANOTHER'S STORY

To appreciate story, we must hear it as particular before fitting it too quickly into a generalized theory or framework. We must, in fact, obtain a decent-sized version of the story. A brief interview or interaction yields only one quick scan of the story—a slice of life, nothing more. We must remember how large the story of a 55-year-old man is, for example. Although we can never grasp the whole of it, we must, at the same time, appreciate it for whom the person is. William Carlos Williams, the noted American poet, is quoted as saying: "Who's against shorthand? No one I know. Who wants to be shortchanged? No one I know" (Coles, 1989, p. 29). In this light, if theory is used as a topographical map to chart where the patient is in a process of exploration shared by others, it has value. If, on the other hand, theory is used as a yardstick only to measure "progress" or to move the patient along a narrowly defined trajectory, it is not helpful. We can miss the experience as the patient is living it.

In nursing as in other professions, anecdotal material is often devalued. Data which can be quantified and generalized is held in higher esteem. The most useful aspect of theory is, I hope, to bring it back to the patient—to understand the particular more fully. In presenting at professional conferences, watch or listen to what happens when one illustrates theory with story. The room gets quieter and people tune into the details of the material. Why? First, it bring theory *home*, home to our human, relational lives. Second, story is one of our best and universal ways of communicating with each other (Brody, 1987).

Knowledge and experience are important to understanding story. In our shrinking world understanding of cultural meanings and contexts is essential to good care. Recently, in the clinical agency where I have students, a patient who is a Jehovah's Witness was described in her chart as "hyper-religious." This is a reflection of the writer's story. My knowledge of Jehovah's Witnesses (taught to me by a patient) led me to think: her story is not understood. In her life context her religious practices were congruent with her community. I posed the following question to my students, most of which are Catholic. How do you think Catholics such as your great-grandfathers were viewed in 1880 in Boston by many mainstream Protestant people unknowledgeable about Catholicism? I would guess something like "hyper-religious": wearing beads, medals, cloth badges, having strange food practices, telling others they will burn in hell if they don't convert to Catholicism, and carrying statues of saints through the streets! What we do not understand we must learn to appreciate about the person's story.

TELLING ONE'S STORY

What does a person need to tell their story? They need a voice—the ability to put the story into thoughts that they can speak to another. Belenky et al. (1986), in their book, *Women's Ways of Knowing*, address the importance of metaphors in the development of language in children. Play is our first experience with metaphor. As we do things "like" grown-ups, we play with others which draws out our "voice." Voice is the ability to "bear witness" to your story as you tell it to another.

"Bearing witness" is a familiar term to many people's religious lives and in another spiritual place—Alcoholics Anonymous (AA). The power of bearing witness to others and being the listener in AA is that of voice and story. A wonderful former patient whose son was killed and who is in AA said to me, "When you lecture to an audience I am sure you look out and see interest in their faces. When I take *commitment* in AA I look out and see love in their eyes. It comes from knowing and appreciating my story as they have lived it."

Churchill and Churchill (1982) describe how the telling of story is at once intimate and distancing. It is intimate because it is our personal account but distancing because time has elapsed between our experience and the present moment. The process of narration can be healing. A former patient of mine agreed to share with nursing students her story of a death in her family and her unresolved feelings that led to panic attacks. After the hour, we sat down. She said she had new insights into her story that came from the telling of it. She found it a healing process. As a supervisor of Robert Coles (1989), the child psychiatrist, once put it:

> *Hearing themselves teach you, through their narrations, the patients will learn the lessons a good instructor learns only when he becomes a willing student, eager to be taught.*

Families have stories. Each member has their story. The poet Edward Hirsch (1989) speaks of siblings:

> The story of siblings is the story of childhood
> Experienced separately and together, one tree
> twisting in different directions, root and branches.
> One piece of land, divided up into parcels
> Acres and half acres, parts of a subdivision
> Memories carved out into official and unofficial versions.
> (p. 32)

The "official" version is the shared version. We additionally have our personal version of the story. Each story is an instrument or voice that together make the family's music.

HELPING PATIENTS TELL THEIR STORIES

This developmental process of having a voice continues. In suffering and illness, some patients have difficulty finding their voice with those around them: nurses, family members, and friends. The fear of not being heard, the unspeakable nature of the suffering, the fear of causing others suffering or the newness of the experience can stifle one's voice. This disconnection is part of the experience of suffering.

Since voice develops through metaphor, we can try to help identify appropriate metaphors for our patients. We can look to literature, film, plays—the domain of great story tellers—as a way to find sources of aid in developing their voice.

There are stories of suffering, hardship, and transcendence that will resonate in patients as they see their story reflected in the one before them. In Julia Lane's (1987) words, "we must stand beside the patient in a spirit of compassion and be midwife to the expressions from the patient's soul without fear" (p. 334). As we listen to the patient, so the patient begins to find the voice to speak with others about his or her suffering.

Thus, it is important for us as nurses to be familiar with works from fiction, poetry, drama, music, and religion. How do you find them? Look, watch, and listen. Some are your personal favorites. Ask your patients. They will teach you to help others. Janet Smerke (1989), in *Interdisciplinary Guide to the Literature for Human Caring*, has put together a wonderful resource book. Tillie Olsen's *Tell Me A Riddle* (1960) is a collection of four stories that powerfully convey scenes of motherhood, alcoholism, adolescent awareness, and family distress as characters attempt to define and understand the meaning in their lives. These stories have resonated for many a patient and student alike.

Children's stories and films provide a wonderful shared metaphorical experience for families. The best of children's literature involves a quest of some sort where hardship and suffering must be endured for a cause affecting others and the protagonist grows as a result. *The Neverending Story* (Eichinger & Deiter, 1984) is one such film with many messages for us all. The main character, a young boy whose mother dies, attempts to cope with his grief privately by reading. He reads a special story in which he becomes a part of it. His is an exploration of uncharted territories. He must cross the swamps of sadness that will drown him if he loses hope and pass through many gates where he must look inward to succeed. He does overcome adversity and learns about himself and those he cares about. Another children's film, *The Land Before Time* (Bluth et al., 1989), has a similar theme. In this film, the spirit of a little dinosaur's dead mother stays with him as he struggles to find his way to a new home.

Recently, while attending a performance of *Les Miserables*, I heard people in the audience around me sobbing. It was the sound of the story on stage resonating poignantly in the hearts of the audience. Perhaps the audience found in the play a measure of their own lives. *Les Miserables* is also a play of suffering, hardship, and hope.

Your patients will give you gifts of metaphors. Here are two given to me:

A young woman who had been sexually abused for years as a child held onto this metaphor, given to her by another patient. "This suffering is like an infected wound. If you stick a bandaid on it, cover it, it will only fester. If you look at it, clean it, let it into the light, it will heal. Yes, it hurts to clean it, and it will leave a scar forever. But remember, scars don't hurt."

And another:

Depression is like being in a big bowl of jello. Every time you've almost climbed to the rim, you slide back down.

I gave this patient the following thought to add:

Look up around the rim. We are here extending our hands out to you. But you must reach up to us if we are to help.

NURSES' STORIES

Story is not solely in the domain of the patient and his or her family. We each have our own story, and it colors how we hear others. We bring to the patient our accumulation of professional and personal education and experiences, those experiences complete with interpreted meanings that are, for each of us, unique. Think of how you are "with" your patients today compared to five or ten years ago. Our stories change, and it influences our ability to hear the story of others. Almost seventeen years ago, as a newly practicing psychiatric nurse, I rarely asked my patients about sexual abuse in their history—and they didn't offer it. Then came graduate school three years later and an influential teacher, Ann Burgess. Learning from my teacher, my readings, my supervisor, and my patients, I was willing and tuned in to hear, and patients told me. They even offered it without being asked. As one family therapist so aptly put it, "When I learn something new, it's as if my patients get mental telegrams letting them know it's okay to tell me this piece of their story now." What is going on here? One's story is ever changing. It is not a static thing. Each day, each encounter colors it.

As patients, nurses also need metaphors. Films, stories, and plays all have their place in our professional lives. They can contribute to our awareness of suffering and compassion. To lecture or read about grief leaves one impression; to see *The Neverending Story* leaves another.

TEACHING STUDENTS TO VALUE STORIES

In education, we need to pay attention to stories—our own and our students'. All nurses bring their stories to the profession. Students, however, learn by knowing what it is to be heard. How can we do this? Faculty can ask students to write down whatever part of their story they would like to share at the beginning of each clinical rotation. With every lecture, whatever the topic, ask students for personal stories that are relevant. For example, in a lecture on seizure disorders, two students described the experience of being very young and observing a seizure in a relative.

A way to bring metaphor into teaching is to begin class with a poem on the subject. Just as we model caring, we can model the use of story and metaphor for students so that they will bring it to their patients.

THE STORY OF NURSING

It is important for students and practicing nurses to look at our stories and consider how they will merge with the story of nursing. Students can be encouraged to envision themselves as part of a long chain of caring, rich in history, that they will pass on to others as we have passed it on to them. We also can view the care we give as part of a chain or circle of caring the patient receives and that each link must be strong and good.

Finding ways to give voice to the stories of nursing is important to the profession. "Pathways to Career Success" was a Sigma Theta Tau chapter program in which ten nurse leaders told their stories. Interestingly, the panelists all commented that preparing to tell their story was an experience full of new awareness about where they are and what contributed to their pathway. Schorr and Zimmerman's (1988) book, *Making Choices, Taking Chances*, is a wonderful compendium in which national nursing leaders tell their stories. They are all instructive and inspirational.

ONE FAMILY'S STORY

Now I will tell you a story. Until diagnosis, this young family had limited experience with suffering or hardship. Then, Linda, the 40-year-old mother was diagnosed with metastatic breast cancer; the family recoiled and could not reframe the family story to include this. No one had a voice to speak to the suffering at hand. Mother, angry with her lot, but well aware of her path, wanted to talk about exploring the road ahead. As an athletic family, they prized the metaphor of sports: "Life is a game, you have to win." Linda needed resources to find her voice and so, as a nurse and long-time friend, I became, in Lane's words, her midwife. Many hours of talk ensued. Bringing her books that spoke of suffering and sharing a journal filled with poems, quotations, and stories all helped her find her voice. She asked me to be present as she asked her husband, Michael, to hear and acknowledge her prognosis and not to see her as "walking away from the game" if she declined chemotherapy. His fierce love for her was making it so hard for him to let her go. She asked him to be on her team and not her opponent.

Weekly facial and foot massages gave comfort to Linda as she became more physically debilitated. This was a particularly helpful method for pouring energy into her spirit.

In finding meaning in her suffering, Linda worked on a spiritual path and on helping her children. *The Neverending Story* and *The Land Before Time* gave her youngest son a metaphor to express his feelings of fear of loss and abandonment with Linda. The films also spoke to her spirit being present with them always.

The Home Planet (Kelley, 1988) is a book of photographs of earth from space with profound poetic quotes by astronauts from around the world. This book also helped Linda on her quest for meaning in her life in the universe.

Each week her friends made the Toll House cookies she could no longer bake for her children. When her father was hospitalized with lung cancer, I went to give the back rub she would have done, were she able.

As the illness progressed, the family needed help to understand her cognitive impairment due to hypercalcemia and morphine. Her physical care needs increased requiring personal nursing care that became a sacred experience to savor.

Her son stole micro machine cars from his favorite cousin. The family needed help to understand his story and this expression of feeling something *more* important that was being stolen from him.

Her death came finally and her funeral, but they were not the end of her story. Friends continued to keep the goodness of her story alive. They gave the family a book filled with memories of shared experiences with Linda. They built and dedicated a playground in her memory at the primary school where she once taught.

Linda's story has been shared with students in classes on separation anxiety, grief, cancer, and family process. Several students were saddened by the news of her death, although they had never met her, but only knew her story. This is still a little part of the *whole* story.

Much like *The Neverending Story*, we become part of the other's story and they part of ours. As it says in the children's book, *In The Night Kitchen*, "I'm in the milk and the milk's in me" (Sendak, 1970, p. 10). We sign up for the ride with all its risks and gifts.

CONCLUSION

Story is the way we come to understand fully another's lived experience. As we approach the patient as compassionate healer, the importance of the patient being able to tell his or her story and the nurse to understand it is clear. By appreciating the need for voice and the value of metaphor and by calling on resources to share with patients in their effort to give voice to their story, we give care of the first order. We also must pay attention to our stories, both personal and professional, for they enhance the care we give others.

REFERENCES

Belenky, M., Clinchy, B., Goldberger, N., & Tarule, J. (1986). *Women's ways of knowing*. New York: Basic Books.

Benner, P., & Wrubel, J. (1989). *The primacy of caring*. Menlo Park, CA: Addison-Wesley.

Bluth, D., Goldman, G., & Pomeroy, J. (Producers). Bluth, D. (Director). *The land before time*. [video cassette] 1989. Universal City, CA: MCA Home Video.

Brody, H. (1987). *Stories of sickness*. New Haven: Yale University Press.

Buber, M. (1958). *I and thou*. New York: Macmillan.

Cassel, E. J. (1982). The nature of suffering and the goals of medicine. *New England Journal of Medicine, 19*, 338–343.

Churchill, L., & Churchill, S. (1982). Storytelling in the medical arenas: The art of self-determination. *Literature and Medicine*, 73–79.

Coles, R. (1989). *The call of the stories*. Boston: Houghton Mifflin.

Cousins, N. (1989). *Head first: the biology of hope*. New York: E.P. Dutton.

Eichinger, B., & Geissler, D. (Producers). Wolfgang, P. (Director). *The neverending story*. [video cassette] 1984. Burbank, CA: Warner Communications.

Gadow, S. (1990, April). *Beyond dualism: The dialectic of caring and knowing*. Paper presented at the Caring and the Compassionate Healer Conference, University of Texas Health Science Center, Houston, Texas.

Hirsch, E. (1989). *The night parade.* New York: Alfred Knopf.

Kelley, K. (Ed.) (1988). *The home planet.* Reading, MA: Addison-Wesley.

Lane, J. (1987). The care of the human spirit. *Journal of Professional Nursing, 3,* 332–337.

Olsen, T. (1961). *Tell me a riddle.* New York: Doubleday.

Roach, Sr. S. (1987). *The human act of caring.* Ottawa: Canadian Hospital Association.

Schorr, T., & Zimmerman, A. (1988). *Making choices, taking chances.* St. Louis: C.V. Mosby.

Sendack, M. (1970). *In the night kitchen.* New York: Harper & Row.

Smerke, J. (1989). *Interdisciplinary guide to literature for human caring.* New York: National League for Nursing.

Watson, J. (1988). *Nursing: Human science and human care.* New York: National League for Nursing.

9

Nurse–Patient Caring: Challenging Our Conventional Wisdom

Kathleen L. Valentine

PROBLEM

Our society is increasingly moving to a human service economy. As it does so, the need to define and value human behaviors provided as a service commodity will increase. As the largest group of health care providers in the second largest industry in the nation, nursing has the potential to greatly influence which aspects of its practice will be rewarded within a service economy. Because "caring is the essence and central focus of nursing practice" (Leininger, 1984) nursing has the responsibility to articulate, measure, and value it. Failure to do so will leave caring as an undervalued aspect of the emerging economic and societal structure.

Traditionally, empirical measurement has been used to inform society and decision makers about phenomena of interest. Policy makers are interested in defining units of production within a service economy. Knowledge obtained through scientific inquiry will be used to define these units of service and will help to determine how resources are allocated. Because of this relationship between scientific inquiry and resource allocation, the scientific questions we choose to research become political decisions (House, 1980). Consequently, our methods of inquiry and the standards used to judge their quality also become political as well as technical issues. For nursing to advance caring, it must also advance the empirical measurement of caring in a way that withstands the scrutiny of the scientific community.

Within the scientific community are long standing traditions and debates about the relative rigor of different modes of inquiry, and what should serve as the standard for quality research. Randomized, experimental design is no longer viewed as the *sine qua non*. Polarized positions about the superiority or inferiority of naturalistic inquiry versus positivism is giving way to a new pragmatism that recognizes the value of both (Cook, 1985; Cronbach, 1980; Patton, 1978). The challenge now is to use the right methods to answer the right questions (Guba & Lincoln, 1981; Patton, 1987). As such, researchers are free to use both qualitative and quantitative methods (Greene, Caracelli, & Graham, 1989; Patton, 1987) and multiple measures (Campbell & Fiske, 1959; Cook, 1985), triangulating the data in a manner to strengthen the inferences that can be drawn from the obtained data (Denzin, 1978; Greene et al., 1989; Patton, 1987; Trochim, 1985). The validity of these empirical measures are then determined by an "integrated evaluative judgment of the degree to which empirical evidence and theoretical rationales support the adequacy and appropriateness of inferences and actions based on test scores or other modes of assessment" (Messick, 1989, p.13). What is validated is not an instrument, test, or observation device but the inferences that emerge from the interpretation of data obtained from the instruments.

These developments within the scientific community present certain challenges to the measurement of caring. What are the right questions? What are the right methods to answer these questions? A researcher has the responsibility to choose an approach which is technically correct, provides useful information, and adequately represents phenomena of interest (Valentine, 1988). To date, the conceptual domain for the phenomenon of caring has not been fully defined. For example, we have no universal meaning or definition of caring, or nurse caring. Caring can be experienced as a moral ideal (Watson, 1985) or as culturally context-specific behaviors Leininger (1986). In addition, practicing nurses have reported evidence of their inability to be caring through such comments as "I'm so busy I don't have time to sit down and talk with the patient." Yet some patients have reported that they don't want or need a nurse to sit with them or hold their hand as an indication of caring (Valentine, 1989a). So what is caring?

The current state of research on theories of caring suggests that caring is context-specific and its universal meaning is still emerging (Leininger, 1988; Stevenson & Tripp-Reimer, 1990). The questions that are asked focus on the discovery and definition of the nature of caring. This suggests that naturalistic approaches which explore caring's context-specific, complex meaning, and define its patterns of relationships are more appropriate than hypotheses testing approaches. Within this naturalistic approach, both quantitative and qualitative methods can be used to describe the phenomenon and its relationships. However, in keeping with naturalistic inquiry, one must stay as close to the phenomenon as possible in order to define and understand it.

To the degree that quantitative measures stay close to a phenomenon, their data can be informative and consistent with naturalistic inquiry. Often, quantitative measurement instruments are used to collect aggregate data. Results are then expressed through descriptive statistics such as averages. In this way patterns of similarity for a group are conveyed. However, quantitative data can be collected so as to express individual differences. Collecting and analyzing data as close to the source as possible helps to preserve the measurement of differences as well as similarities. This study used quantitative methods both in the aggregate and individualized for nurse–patient pairs. This was done because caring is an interactive process that occurs between persons. In order to study nurse–patient caring, the researcher must measure the lived experiences of caring between nurses and patients within specific shared caring encounters. The data collected within this study—from one hospital setting—satisfies this requirement.

PURPOSE

In this paper, I will describe the application of multiple measures and methods as part of a naturalistic study of caring, which explores how nurses and patients viewed the phenomenon of caring as it occurred within specific encounters. *Congruence* here is defined as the agreement between each nurse–patient pair about their perceptions of caring during a specific encounter.

Specifically, this paper will address the following areas related to nurse–patient caring:

1. How was congruence conceptualized and measured within this study?

2. What was the congruence between nurse–patient pairs in specific encounters?

3. How well did the aggregate and the individualized quantitative measures represent the conceptualized concept of congruence?

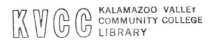

4. To what degree did the quantitative measures of congruence correspond with the qualitative responses given by the nurse–patient pairs?

METHODOLOGY

The Conceptualization of Congruence

Past conceptualizations of caring have included phenomenological studies
describing the lived experiences of caring (Aamodt et al., 1984; Boyle, 1984;
Brown, 1986; Gaut, 1984; Leininger, 1981a, b, 1986; Ray, 1981; Riemen, 1986).
Less frequently, quantitative measures have been used to explore the meaning
of caring (Gardner & Wheeler, 1981; Larson, 1987; Mayer, 1987). In studies
in which quantitative methods were used, the data were examined in the
aggregate and were not matched with specific nurse–patient respondent pairs.

For this study, the measurement of congruence occurred within the context
of a larger study. The larger study used a naturalistic approach to define caring
and its relationship to productivity and health outcomes variables (Valentine,
1989b). Within the larger study the conceptual domain of caring was specified
through the use of multiple measures and methods (Valentine, 1989a, 1989b,
1989c). Based on the data from the domain specification phase of the study, two
Likert-type questionnaires were developed. Both the Nurse Caring Questionnaire (NCQ) and the Patient Caring Questionnaire (PCQ) had 61 items which
were identical except for pronoun reference. The questionnaires measured the
presence of caring which had occurred between specific nurse–patient pairs on a
particular shift. The total score for each patient and each nurse represented
their perception of the *presence* of caring as a whole.

The measure of congruence calculated for this study measured questionnaire item responses for the matched nurse–patient pair. It was designed to
measure the degree to which the nurse–patient pair agreed about the specific
aspects of caring which had occurred between them as represented by the
61 items on the questionnaire. It has greater specificity than the total scores
calculated for the NCQ and PCQ. Examples of questionnaire items and the
formula for the calculation of congruence are included in Table 9–1.

Sample

Ninety-one hysterectomy patients and their nurses each completed a 61-
item, Likert-type questionnaire which measured the degree to which caring

Table 9–1

PCQ					
The nurse who cared for me on this shift today treated me with:					
Kindness	1	2	3	4	5
Respect	1	2	3	4	5
Empathy	1	2	3	4	5
NCQ					
As I cared for this patient today I was able to treat her with:					
Kindness	1	2	3	4	5
Respect	1	2	3	4	5
Empathy	1	2	3	4	5

Congruence Calculation—Based on SPSSX statistical package.
Compute Nmean = mean (N10 to N61)
Compute Pmean = mean (PT10 to PT61)
Compute NSD = SD (N10 to N61)
Compute PSD = SD (PT10 to PT61)
Do repeat R = R10 to R61/N = N10 to N61/P = PT10 to PT61
If (NSD GT O and PSD GT O) R = (N-Nmean)* (P-Pmean)/(NSD*PSD)
End repeat
Compute Rmean = mean (R10 to R61)

*Asterisk means multiply by.

occurred in specific nurse–patient encounters. These data were collected over a six-month period in one acute-care hospital setting.

Several types of data were collected from each nurse–patient pair, three of which will be discussed here. Each nurse completed a NCQ and each patient completed a PCQ. In addition, each respondent was asked to write a narrative about what had occurred within that encounter. In this way, quantitative and qualitative data were both collected from each pair.

Figure 9-1 shows the response rate for these respondents. Each nurse and patient completed and mailed their questionnaires separately. Therefore, the responses for the NCQ and PCQ were not always received as a matched pair. Consequently, there were different sample sizes for the different analyses performed. Finally, not all respondents wrote a narrative, and some who did returned nonuseable questionnaire responses. For data which was received, three different sets of analyses were performed:

1. Aggregate: Total scores for NCQ and PCQ (N = 72 NCQ; N = 78 PCQ) This measured the presence of caring.

2. Matched Pair: Nurse-patient pair (N = 59 NCQ/PCQ pair) This measured congruence.

3. Qualitative responses (N = 51) This provided information to help understand the other two measures.

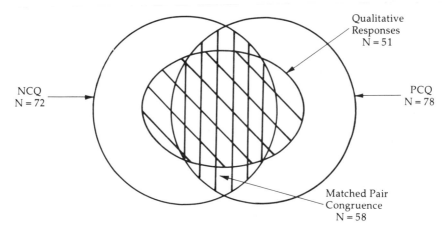

Figure 9-1

Data Collection

Patients who entered the hospital for preadmission testing for hysterectomy surgery were informed about the research study on caring. Each woman was asked to sign a permission form in which she agreed to complete questionnaires while in the hospital and which allowed the investigator to review her medical record. Each nurse in the study consented to complete a questionnaire for each participating patient for whom she provided nursing care.

The NCQ and PCQ questionnaires were attached to the medical record. The questionnaires were administered to the patient and the nurse when the patient stopped intramuscular pain medication. This was usually on the third post-operative day. At the end of the shift, the nurse completed the NCQ and the patient completed the PCQ. Each questionnaire was then sealed in an envelope by the respondent and mailed to the investigator.

ANALYSIS AND RESULTS

Congruence Between Nurses and Patients

The congruence score was calculated by computing for each pair of nurse-patient respondents correlations of paired questionnaire items. The individual paired item correlations were then averaged to derive a congruence score (see Table 9-1). For this measure, high positive correlation represented agreement and high negative correlations represented disagreement. Illustrations of this can be seen in Table 9-2. A congruence score of .56 is found for the nurse-patient pair for Patient #91. This represents moderate agreement for that pair about the specific and positive aspects of caring which occurred between them. If a nurse-patient pair had a congruence score of −.71, then it would represent strong negative agreement that caring was absent. Similarly, a congruence score of .91 would represent a strong positive agreement about the specific and positive presence of caring.

Congruence scores ranged between −.07 and .60. The mean correlation for the total group of matched nurse-patient pairs was quite low (.18). This suggests that for a given paired nurse-patient encounter there was little congruence between nurses' and patients' caring scores; they neither agreed nor disagreed about the caring which occurred in a given encounter.

A factor affecting these scores will be discussed in the section on the quality of data.

Presence of Caring as Measured by Aggregate Data

The mean score for nurses on the NCQ was 209, representing 80 percent of the total possible score. The mean score for patients on the PCQ was 205, representing 79 percent of the total possible score. Table 9-2 displays the patient responses in four categories: low (scores between 52–195), medium (scores between 196–233), high (scores between 234–260), and "missing." These groupings will be further discussed in the section on triangulation of the data.

Comparison of Aggregate and Matched Pair Responses

In the aggregate, there was a significant but low-moderate relationship between the patients' and nurses' total questionnaire scores. (correlation of .31, $(p < .05)$. This is in contrast to the congruence score which was based on *paired item scores*, and had a correlation of .18 indicating little congruence. While these total score correlations are statistically significant, neither the total caring score nor the congruence score indicate strong relationships between nurses' and patients' perceptions of caring.

The congruence score and the total NCQ and PCQ scores were not significantly correlated. This finding suggests that the congruence score is measuring

Table 9–2

Comparison of Aggregate Patient Caring Scores, Congruence and Narrative

Aggregate Patient Caring Questionnaire

Low: Scores 52–195			Medium: Scores 196–233		
Patient ID	Congruence Score	Presence of Narrative	Patient ID	Congruence Score	Presence of Narrative
8			2	.10	– N
9	.40	– P	7		
11			10		+ P
		+ N –			– N
12	–.05		20	.02	– P
		– N	22		
14	.23	+ P +	23		
15			24		
25	.33	– P	29		+ P
26		– P	35	.37	+ P
27	–.07	– P	36		
		+ N –	40		
33	.27		42		
34			50		
39	.20	– P	51		– P
		– N	53		
49	.35		55		
55			56		
56		+ P –	58		
68			60	.08	+ P –
72		– P	65		
74		– P	69		
77	.05	+ P –	79		
82			86	.06	+ P
84			89		
85	.03	– P			
88	.09	+ P –			
91	.56	+ P –			

Percent of Patients with Written Comments: 61%   Percent of Patients with Written Comments: 29%

High: Scores 234–260			Missing Data		
Patient ID	Congruence Score	Presence of Narrative	Patient ID	Congruence Score	Presence of Narrative
5	.00	– N	4		+ P
16	.23	+ P	6		
17	– .02	+ P	13		+ N
		+ N –	30		

TABLE 9–2 (continued)

Patient ID	Congruence Score	Presence of Narrative	Patient ID	Congruence Score	Presence of Narrative
18	.01	+ P	32	.06	+ P
19	.41	+ P +	38		+ P
21	.22	+ P	43		– P
37		+ P	45		
41		+ P	47	.14	+ P –
44		+ P	61		
48		+ P –	62	.19	+ P –
52			70		– P
54	.60	+ P	73	.03	– P
59		+ P			
63		+ P –			
64					
65					
67		+ P			
78					
87	.24	+ P –			

Percent of Patients with Written Comments: 74%	Percent of Patients with Written Comments: 69%

Key: + P = Positive Patient Comments
+ N = Positive Nursing Comments
– P = Negative Patient Comments
– N = Negative Nursing Comments
+ – = Mixed Comments

something separate from the total caring scores. It is measuring the degree to which matched pairs of nurses and patients agree about specific aspects of caring based on questionnaire items rather than total scores.

In conclusion, there is some evidence for agreement between nurses and patients about the presence of caring when measured in the aggregate. However, when congruence was figured on an item-for-item basis for each matched pair in the nurse–patient encounter, then there was less evidence of agreement or disagreement between nurses and patients about what occurred. This suggests that more clarification between nurses and patients is necessary about what the important aspects of caring are so that, within specific encounters, carative aspects of the relationship can be enhanced. Presumably, the greater the congruence in beliefs between caregiver and care receiver, the greater the opportunity for healing.

DISCUSSION

The Quality of the Data

Based on the findings above, there is support for the premise that aggregate quantitative data reflect different aspects of a phenomenon than do the matched pair data. Which of these measures more adequately represents the phenomenon? Are the two approaches measuring different phenomena? Or are they measuring different dimensions of the same phenomenon of caring?

In the aggregate, the total scores for the NCQ and PCQ had Cronbach's alpha internal consistency reliability estimates of .99 each. This suggests that the questionnaires were reliably measuring some common phenomenon. Additionally, both nurses and patients measured moderately high levels for the presence of caring (79 percent and 80 percent). This suggests that in the aggregate both nurses and patients agreed that caring was present in their encounters.

However, these aggregate measures of caring also revealed differences in the way that nurses and patients answered the questionnaire. In general, when answering the Likert-type questionnaire responses, patients had more variance in their responses than did the nurses. Most nurses' answers ranged between 3 (neither agree/nor disagree) to 5 (strongly agree); while patients used the full range of responses, from 1 (strongly disagree) to 5 (strongly agree).

This restricted range of responses for nurses affected correlations and other relational analyses. When there is little variance in responses, then it is more difficult to show relationships. This restricted range problem could have been due to nurses' using the scale in a different way than patients. The factors contributory to the nurses' using only the top part of the range also could have been due to social desirability and socialization to the professional nursing role, in which anything less than excellence is considered unacceptable. That is, the nurses may have found it difficult to evaluate any aspect of their care as below average, thus they did not use the lower end of the rating scale. Patients, as recipients of caring, did not harbor such restrictions and thus used the full range of responses. Therefore, while difference in use of the scale may be a measurement artifact, it also may represent some of the cultural incongruities of caring between professional nurses and clients which Leininger (1981b) has discussed.

This restricted response range for nurses also affected the quality of the congruence measure. In computing the congruence score, all cases in which there was no variance in item responses for either the nurse or the patient were deleted. This then dropped 13 cases in which the patient or nurse answered all questions with the same response, reducing the pool of available matched pairs from 58 to 45, and also reducing the confidence with which this measure can be used because of the small sample size. This measure may be underestimating the amount of agreement between nurses and patients because of the need to drop cases which had no variance questionnaire item responses. On the other hand, the 13 dropped cases may represent those patients or nurses who did not answer the questionnaire seriously. There is no way to resolve this question from the data.

What is apparent from the data is that aggregate quantitative measures and the encounter-specific congruence scores provide different but related information. Do the measures accurately reflect an actual lack of congruence between nurse and patient perceptions of caring, or are there measurement artifacts which interfere with the ability to reveal congruence which exists, but can't be measured? To explore this issue, analyses of qualitative responses that accompanied the questionnaires were performed.

Triangulation of Qualitative and Quantitative Measures

The focus of this paper thus far has emphasized the nurse and patient quantitative measures both in the aggregate and as measured by congruence. Yet how well does the narrative portion of the questionnaire correspond with the quantitative findings? Table 9-2 shows the breakdown of patient scores and an analysis of whether or not the accompanying narrative was positive, negative, or mixed in relation to perceptions of nurse caring.

In the triangulation of data, the researcher looks for patterns of convergence which help to confirm findings inferred from other data. In this case, the qualitative responses show some pattern on the aggregate level, but do not show a consistent pattern as it relates to the congruence score.

On the aggregate level, more patients wrote narrative comments than did nurses. Also, the patients who scored on the extremes for the patient caring questionnaire (PCQ) wrote more narrative comments than the patients in the middle. Sixty-one percent of patients with "low" scores, 29 percent with "medium" scores, and 74 percent with "high" scores had narrative data present. Comments in the lower scores tended to be negative. Conversely, the "high" scoring group tended to be positive about the quality of nurse caring. These comments also included suggestions about how to improve the system so that the nurse could be even more caring. For the middle group of patients, only 25 percent wrote narrative comments. Thus, the patients on the extremes tended to comment on their care while the patients in the middle did not.

There was another group of patient–nurse pairings which deserves comment. These were the "missing data" group. For this group, no total PCQ score could be calculated because some items were not answered. Despite this, for some of these nurse–patient pairs, congruence scores could be calculated because missing data in this method was dealt with differently. In this group of patients and nurses, there were often long narratives explaining their perceptions of care.

For the congruence score, there were no outstanding patterns of correspondence between the calculated congruence score and the total patient score. It was not true that the higher the congruence score, the higher the overall patient score. Nor was it true that the higher the congruence score, the more likely there was to be a positive comment. What was true, however, was that if a congruence score could be calculated, there was likely to be some narrative comment.

Therefore, the qualitative data supported the aggregate data findings to some extent. The higher the total score, the more likely that the narrative would be present and positive. This provides information for convergent validity of the aggregate measures of caring. However, it neither confirms nor denies the validity of the congruence measure. It shows no pattern. This is one of the challenges in triangulation of data. Clear convergence or divergence helps to build a case for, or against, a finding. A nonrelationship leaves us searching for another avenue of corroborative evidence for validity. However, one study or program of research cannot provide all the necessary information for validation (Messick, 1989). Other studies in different settings, and with different populations, will need to be conducted to further explore this issue.

ISSUES AND FUTURE IMPLICATIONS

Congruence was conceptualized as the correlation between nurse–patient pair responses to items on a Likert-type questionnaire. It was measured quantitatively for specific nurse–patient pairs in specific encounters. Using this measure, congruence was low (.18). It is not known if the measurement artifacts described in this paper (restricted range, dropping cases) prevented adequate representation of congruence which existed; or conversely, if the measures accurately represented a lack of congruence between nurses and patients. Although caring as a whole was seen as present in nurse–patient encounters, specific dimensions of caring were not identical.

Qualitative response to the questionnaire did not help to definitively sort out a pattern of responses relative to congruence and the total perception of caring. The exception to this was that patients on the extremes (scoring high or low on the total questionnaire) tended to enrich their responses with narrative. In general nurses used narrative responses sparingly. A second interesting aspect of the comparison of qualitative and quantitative data collection is that so many of the "missing data" group wrote extensive narrative comments. This indicates that despite being dropped from quantitative analyses, these persons certainly were active participants in the study. They wanted their voice to be heard. Such richness of information obtained from the use of mixed methods argues for continued use of multiple methods and measures to inform us about phenomenon.

Caring is a complex phenomenon, its mysteries as a human mode of being will not be able to be revealed through empirical research alone, no matter how elegant our methods, measures, or analyses. The presence of these limitations does not rule out the ability to explore some of caring's dimensions, particularly those related to professional nurse caring. It is the profession's responsibility to continue to rise to the challenge of articulating its scope of practice and responsibilities. Caring, as a central focus of nursing, must be researched. In the search for caring's meaning and relevance in today's health care system, both quantitative and qualitative methods will prove to be invaluable techniques for contributing to our knowledge.

REFERENCES

Aamodt, A., Grassl-Herwehe, S., Farrell, F., & Hutter, J. (1984). The child's view of chemically induced alopecia. In M. M. Leininger (Ed.), *Care: The essence of nursing and health* (pp. 217–231). Thorofare, NJ: Slack.

Boyle, J. (1984). Indigenous caring practices in a Guatemalan Colonia. In M. M. Leininger (Ed.), *Care: The essence of nursing and health* (pp. 123–132). Thorofare, NJ: Charles B. Slack Incorporated.

Brown, L. (1986). The experience of care: Patient perspective. In Z. R. Wolf (Ed.), *Topics in clinical nursing*. Aspen, CO: Aspen Publishers.

Campbell, D. T., & Fiske, D. W. (1959). Convergent and discriminant validation by the multitrait-multimethod Matrix. *Psychological Bulletin, 56*(2), 81–105.

Cook, T. D. (1985). Postpositivist critical multiplism. In R. Shotland & M. Mark (Eds.), *Social science and social policy* (pp. 21–62). Beverly Hills: Sage.

Cronbach, L. J. (1980). *Toward reform of program evaluation*. San Francisco: Jossey-Bass.

Denzin, N. K. (1978). The logic of naturalistic inquiry. In N. K. Denzin (Ed.), *Sociological methods: A sourcebook.* New York: McGraw Hill.

Gardner, K., & Wheeler, E. (1981). Patients' and staff nurses' perceptions of supportive nursing behaviors: A preliminary analysis. In M. M. Leininger (Ed.), *Caring: An essentiaal human need* (pp. 109–113). New Jersey: Charles B. Slack.

Gaut, D. A. (1984). A theoretic description of caring as action. In M. M. Leininger (Ed.), *Care: The essence of nursing and health* (pp. 27–44). Thorofare, NJ: Slack.

Greene, J., Caracelli, V., & Graham W. (1989). Toward a conceptual framework for mixed-method evaluation. *Educational Evaluation and Policy Analysis, 7*(3), 255–74.

Guba, E., & Lincoln, Y. (1981). *Effective evaluation.* San Francisco: Jossey-Bass.

House, E. R. (1980). *Evaluating with validity.* Beverly Hills: Sage.

Larson, P. J. (1987). Comparison of cancer patients' and professional nurses' perceptions of important nurse caring behaviors. *Heart and Lung, 16*(2), 187–192.

Leininger, M. M. (1981a). The phenomenon of caring: Importance, research questions, and theoretical considerations. In M. M. Leininger (Ed.), *Care: An essential human need* (pp. 3–15).

Leininger, M. M. (1981b). Some philosophical, historical, and taxonomic aspects of nursing and caring in the American Culture. In M. M. Leininger (Ed.), *Care: An essential human need* (pp.133–143). Thorofare, NJ: Charles B. Slack.

Leininger, M. M. (1984). Care: The essence of nursing and health. In M. M. Leininger (Ed.), *Care: The essence of nursing and health* (pp. 3–15). Thorofare, NJ: Charles B. Slack.

Leininger, M. M. (1986). Care facilitation and resistance factors in the culture of nursing. *Topics in Clinical Nursing, 8*(2), 1–12.

Leininger, M. M. (1988). History, issues and trends in the discovery and uses of care in nursing. In M. M. Leininger (Ed.), *Care: Discovery and uses in clinical and community nursing* (pp. 11–28). Detroit: Wayne State Press.

Mayer, D. K. (1987). Oncology nurses' versus patients' perceptions of nurses caring behaviors: A replication study. *Oncology Nursing Forum, 14*(3), 48–52.

Messick, S. (1989). Validity. In R. Linn (Ed.), *Educational measurement* (pp. 13–104). New York: Macmillan Publishing.

Patton, M. Q. (1978). *Utilization-focused evaluation.* Beverly Hills: Sage.

Patton, M. Q. (1987). *How to use qualitative methods in evaluation.* Newbury Park, CA: Sage Publications.

Ray, M. A. (1981). A study of caring within an institutional culture. *Dissertation Abstracts International, 42*(06), 2310.

Riemen, D. J. (1986). Noncaring and caring in the clinical setting: Patients' descriptions. *Topics in Clinical Nursing 8*(2), 30–36.

Stevenson, J., & Tripp-Reimer, T. (1990). J. Stevenson & T. Tripp-Reimer (Eds.), *Knowledge about care and caring: State of the art and future developments.* Proceedings of the Wingspread Conference, February 1–3, 1989. Kansas City: American Academy of Nursing.

Trochim, W. (1985). Pattern matching, validity, and conceptualization in program evaluation. *Evaluation Review 9*, 575–604.

Valentine, K. (1988). Advancing care and ethics in health management: An evaluation strategy. In M. M. Leininger (Ed.), *Care: Discovery and uses in clinical and community nursing* (pp. 151–168). Detroit: Wayne State Press.

Valentine, K. (1989a). Contributions to the theory of care. *Evaluation and Program Planning, 12*(1), 17–24.

Valentine, K. (1989b). The value of caring nurses: Implications for patient satisfaction, quality of care and cost. *University Microfilms International* (University Microfilms No. 9001333).

Valentine, K. (1989c). Caring is more than kindness: Modeling its complexities. *Journal of Nursing Administration, 19*(11), 28–34.

Watson, J. (1985). *Nursing: Human science and human care.* Connecticut: Appleton-Century-Crofts.

Weiss, C. J. (1988). Model to discover, validate, and use care in nursing. In M. M. Leininger (Ed.), *Care: Discovery and uses in clinical and community nursing* (pp. 139–150). Detroit: Wayne State Press.

10

I Sent Myself a Card Today

Doris S. Greiner
Nassif J. Cannon

The message of and about caring in this paper begins with a story. We are a nurse and a physician who see patients in a medicine clinic within the county hospital located in a large southern city. Though life threatening illnesses are part of the experience of some of the patients, most individuals seen in the clinic are experiencing major difficulties in living. Medical symptoms are one part of a complex of ongoing troubles. One experience, contained in the following story, prompted us both to think about caring from a different perspective. Our story and the stories of the patients are told from the perspective of the nurse.

On the day before Thanksgiving I entered a patient room of an indigent care hospital to see a woman who had been admitted for asthma. I had seen this woman once in the outpatient clinic, approximately two months previously. As she spoke about herself and her situation, conveying an inescapable loneliness, she shifted focus to indicate a greeting card on the tray table over the foot of her bed. I was suddenly aware of the drabness of the room, everywhere variations on a shade of grey except for the brightness in the card. As I became thus aware, she said, "I sent myself a card today."

She and I went on to talk for a few more minutes. She continued to want her parents and sisters to express interest in her. She had told them that she was in the hospital and they had promised to come visit. No one had come. From her description in our first and only other encounter I remembered that there was a man in her life who "Lets me stay with him." He was too ill to come. She was alone, had asked a nurse to buy the card for her and the nurse had done so. Now she faced the night, and probably the holiday, alone. We focused on relaxation and visualization as ways to be with the period before sleep that night which she was dreading. I left with her words "I sent myself a card today" echoing in my head.

Two thoughts took form as I finished my tasks at the clinic:

1. *This woman had let me know of something I could tangibly do for her.*

2. *More importantly, she had taken action to meet a need from resources within herself.*

I prepared a greeting card for her and asked Nass [Dr. Cannon] to give it to her when making hospital rounds on Thanksgiving Day. His story for me the next Wednesday when I arrived at the clinic was that the patient had been discharged Thanksgiving morning before he arrived. But on Monday she had come to the clinic seeking medication for headache. Though he could not prescribe what she was asking for, he remembered the card, got it for her, and was keenly aware that she left smiling and with no apparent signs of the headache.

Reflecting on this story, we were both aware that we had learned something that might be useful to other patients who come to the clinic. I teach psychiatric-mental health nursing in the graduate program at a university. I have always believed that for me to teach in a practice profession, I would need to be involved in direct practice. This I have done in a family oriented private practice and at a public mental health center. In addition, for the last four years I have spent one afternoon a week in the medicine clinic seeing two to four individuals referred to me by Nass, who is a physician specializing in internal medicine and infectious diseases. Graduate students have also come with me to this setting. This collaborative practice is described in more detail in an article that appeared in *Family Systems Medicine* and authored by Dashiff, Greiner, and Cannon (1990).

My work as a clinical specialist is informed by a theoretic conceptualization of families as emotional systems (Bowen, 1978). In this setting, I attempt to help individuals identify issues in the emotional systems of which they are a part and identify choices in regard to their own part in the situations which they describe. In many situations there seem to be no choices, however, thinking through the experiences they are having can make possibilities apparent that were previously hidden. In doing this work, I believe that it is important for me to be meaningfully connected to the individuals with whom I am working without getting caught in automatic emotional processes that maintain ineffective patterns of behavior. I attempt to help them use their mind to free energy for healing and change. Most basically, I listen to their stories.

When Ms. O said "I sent myself a card today," not only did she communicate her isolation and loneliness, she also provided a therapeutic effort toward a healing of herself and her wounds. In addition, she provided us with another means of relating, communicating, and treating. Her action suggested another exterior action I might use to mirror interior compassionate concern. I began to use cards as a way of making tangible the healing that I believe can come from the talking encounter. I had three images in mind as I proceeded.

1. The beauty of the card I had seen in the hospital room.
2. That of the prescription pad.
3. The words on a card.

It was important to me to reproduce the beauty of the card I had seen. Watson (1987, 1988) reminds us of the crucial value of finding healing metaphors. Finding ways of accessing and being with what we can know from both the right and the left of our experience is captured in the poem she quotes by Marilyn Krysl (1990). That poem begins, "The left hand trails in the water, The right is tying knots." Watson speaks of finding, as did Hildegard of Bingen in the twelfth century, esthetic as well as scientific expression. I chose cards that I found beautiful and that I thought would at minimum bring a small thing of beauty into the day for the patient and thus into both our lives.

The idea of prescription permeates most health care settings. As Nass and I each listen to people at the clinic, we hear them attempting to make sense of what they are experiencing. Though there are themes that recur in the symptom accounts and the stories, each person is unique. However, one thing that they almost certainly have in common is that they leave the clinic with a small piece of paper, that is, a prescription. It is rare to find a set of symptoms for which some pill is not clearly indicated. It is also a direction that we find that both of our minds take in the face of the massive unsolvable problems in living which we hear in this clinic. Providing another form of prescription fit into the setting and fit with our concept of caring.

Thus, I chose to take the focus from my time with the patient into the realm of prescription, that is, something each one might think about further, or do. When I started I thought I would need to come up with some wise formulation. What would the words be? I knew that no easy formula would fit. The words would need to come from what the patient and I had talked about. The first woman to whom I gave a card helped to clarify my thinking about the words.

Three stories related to the use of the cards are examples of our early findings in this effort. The first card I wrote was for a woman recovering from a second serious stroke that left her unable to carry out usual tasks. She gets extremely frustrated and tense and has been making a conscious effort to relax. I wanted to capitalize on something she was already doing and was writing, "Remember to relax, adding an additional session/day," when she said, "I need patience. Put that on there, too." And so I wrote "for you—an abundance of patience." I signed my name on the card and noted the date. Her immediate response was to say that this would go on her refrigerator. Since, she has reported on its daily usefulness although not for any message about relaxation. The intervening sudden death of her husband precluded an attempt on my part to learn in her words an exact meaning the card had for her. In the midst of the other things she talked through, however, I took note of the comment that she looks at the card every day.

A more private use of the card was apparent in the response of the woman who put it into her purse commenting on the importance of keeping it to herself. Two aspects of her action were noteworthy to me. First, in her living situation privacy is not easily come by. A purse can be a single safe place. (One woman carries her phone in her purse so that, when she is away, another family member will not use it for long distance calls.) But the more important reason came from what I consider to be an error on my part. The issue she had been discussing with me was the behavior of her youngest son who had just dropped out of school as he struggles through that long no man's land between childhood and adulthood. The question she and I were addressing— "what does your son need from you at this stage in your lives?"—I put on the card for her further consideration between sessions. She expressed concern that her son might see the card and become angry that she had been talking about him. Though she is aware of the usefulness of talking about a person in preparation for talking to that person and or simply changing her own unconstructive efforts on his behalf, this prescriptive card as an opening to talking with her son was not the point, nor effective. Remembering to focus my statements on the cards to the person with whom I am working was underlined in this interaction.

The third story about the fate of the card emphasized a ripple effect of our encounters: caring extended to other relationships. The woman involved was severely depressed two years ago when she was first seen in the clinic. She has seemingly come to terms with her childless state and the nature of the marriage she is in. She is no longer depressed and has been exploring the basic question, "what next?" She is very heavy and wants to lose weight as she prepares to move out into the bigger world beyond her own home. Her requests for prescription were exercise oriented, and as I wrote she told me to add that she should use the exercise rope, something in the home that I did not even know existed. By this time I had caught the reality that the messages were coming from within the patients; it was my job to listen and to write.

Six weeks later this woman returned to the clinic, having had unexpected gall bladder surgery in the meantime. She spoke of the events surrounding the surgery. As we finished I asked if she had brought the card for me to add today's prescription or did she need a new one. She had not brought it but said she would like to tell me what she did do. Upon returning home six weeks before she had called a sister and told her she needed $25 to fill the prescription she had gotten that day at the clinic. She said, "I never ask for anything so she was surprised but said yes and that she would bring it to church that night." The sister handed the patient a check when she saw her. The patient said, "Maybe you better see the prescription first." After the initial—you tricked me—response, she reported that they agreed this was the best kind of prescription. Not yet finished, she made a similar contact with a brother she sees less often and from whom she is even less likely to ask for something. Once again she learned that the $25 was hers for the asking. This time she took care to say, "You better see the prescription first." I hear in this story so many messages, not the least of which is that she is feeling valuable and valued. As I recall those earlier depressed days when her total message was "I am worthless," the message about her own value sounds even richer and more beautiful in contrast.

In our collaborative work we have taken time at the end of many clinic days to talk to each other. Caring is one among topics that have been examined. Sister Simone Roach (1984) speaks of the five Cs of caring, two of which are *compassion* and *competence*. She says compassion assumes competence. We emphasize this because we do experience it as a given that is too easily overlooked. What is described here presupposes professional competence to intervene with established treatments for particular symptoms. Given that assumption, as we have talked we have affirmed that established treatments are always prescribed within the larger context of patients' lives. Knowing precedes caring. We must be still and silent and receive the stories of the people we see. Knowing them in the context of their woundedness has led us to a compassionate attitude, an attentiveness to the uniqueness of their being in the world. These interior movements within us of knowing and compassion lead us to an exterior action of caring. Caring in this sense is not an interior posture, but an exterior action that mirrors our interior experience.

The implications of this work for health care education, health care delivery, and research follow the same pattern that the use of the cards has followed for us. We start with listening to patients, to all of what they convey, believing their words and symptoms as part of a larger truth, that within each of us energy is available to be freed for healing and health. We proceed to look within for the inner resources that give direction to the external acts, also known as delivery of health care services. When we attempt to educate, patient encounters are the richest focus. The inner resources of the nurse and physician provide the connecting link to the inner resources of the patient. Our research, when it is about human experience, is always a search and never context free.

Our search leads us to a concept of integrative medicine, outlined in Nass' article, *The Broken Healer*, (Cannon, 1987). This concept of health and healing involves a process of progressive reconciliation and integration of body, mind, and soul, not merely the absence of suffering or disease. Health of the body is not only the absence of bodily illness but also reconciliation with mind. The body as subordinated to the governance of right reason becomes disciplined. Hence, one governs what one eats, drinks, and how much exercise one gets. The mind rules the behavior of the body in accord with right reason, seeking for the body that which will bring it health. Similarly the mind governed by the soul seeks healthful knowledge and wisdom. Health of the mind involves a reconciliation of mind to soul. It is possible for one's mind to have unhealthy pursuits. There are deadly things to know, for example, the sadistic knowledge of torturing and killing others. (Some patients who come to this clinic have direct experience with this kind of knowledge.) Our rejection of the knowledge of evil and the pursuit of healthful knowledge and wisdom results in health of mind and reconciliation with soul. Our souls grow in health by the pursuit of a grace-filled life, manifested by love of self and neighbor. Progressive reconciliation and integration of the body, mind, and soul allows a person to grow in health and wholeness.

The philosophy which underlies our approach to providing care is predicated upon the golden rule, treat others as you would want to be treated. We believe this rule offers guidance in our relationships because it recognizes our equality based on our shared humanity. We recognize the other person as a distinct unique individual with a personal history. We recognize their unique individuality as predicated on genetic and environmental factors governing their development. But underlying our distinctions, we believe there is a mutuality and common ground. Apart from sharing in the human race, we occupy a common space and time of encounter. We share common desires, hopes, and expectations. We believe the rule points to an even deeper spiritual reality—the other person is a complimentary part of us. We compliment and complete one another because we share in the mystery of being made in the image and likeness of God. We mirror and convey this image and likeness to one another and in so doing experience others as complimentary persons, necessary for our very own growth in wholeness.

Our perception of effective therapy has much to do with our perception of health and disease. If we limit the perception of health to merely the absence of disease, we limit our perception of therapy to that which eradicates or alleviates disease. Our current medical models do this. They often provide one-dimensional therapy for a one-dimensional perception of health and disease. By contrast, if we perceive health and healing as reconciliation, progressive integration of body, mind, and spirit, we open ourselves to a vast array of possibilities for healing.

Our search to find effective ways of expressing caring continues. The cards are one way, but they don't work in all instances. I have experienced times when connection with the patient was not possible for me, and one way I was aware of it was noting my inability to use the card. Gadow (1990) has talked of nursing as a region of experience and of finding a safe and honorable passage with people. I know that passage to be wonderfully, touchingly apparent at times, and at others totally elusive. At these times I have been effectively reminded to put my left hand back into the water (Krysl, 1980). My search, our search, continues.

REFERENCES

Bowen, M. (1978). *Family therapy in clinical practice.* New York: Jason Aronson.

Cannon, M. J. (1987). The wounded healer. *Humane Medicine, 3*(2), 121–181.

Dashiff, C., Greiner, D. S., & Cannon, N. J. (1990). Physician and nurse collaboration in a medical indigent clinic. *Family Systems Medicine, 8,* 57–70.

Gadow, S. (1990, April). *Beyond dualism: The dialetic of caring and knowing.* Paper presented at the Caring Conference, Houston, TX.

Krysl, M. (1980). Poem for the left and right hand, in *More palamino please, more fuchsia.* Cleveland: Cleveland State University Poetry Center.

Roach, M. S. (1984). *Caring: The human mode of being, implications for nursing* (Perspectives in Caring Monograph 10). Toronto: Faculty of Nursing, University of Toronto.

Watson, J. (1987). Nursing on the caring edge: Metaphorical vignettes. *Advances in Nursing Science, 10*(1), 10–18.

Watson, J. (1988). New dimensions of human caring theory. *Nursing Science Quarterly, 1*(4), 175–181.

11

Caring in Nursing Administration: Healing through Empowering

Carolyn L. Brown

A nurse stands in the middle of the medication room, head lowered, hands clenched at her sides, her face a portrait of anguish as tears stream down her face. The reason? She is "in charge" on a short-staffed evening shift. Several colleagues have called in sick. She is left with the responsibility for the care of all of the patients on her unit, a responsibility usually shared with one or two more colleagues. Frustration, anger, helplessness, and impotence are her feelings. The staffing decisions were made at a higher level of the hierarchy, and she has no control over her situation. She feels bound to care for her clients. After all, were she not there, then who would care for them? She also knows that the care she can give will be incomplete, and in her eyes, inadequate. Equally important, she believes no one in the hospital hierarchy cares for her. No one asks her to participate in the decisions affecting her or her practice. No one values her input. She feels overpowered.

Nurse administrators, working in a health care environment with constrained resources, make decisions affecting nurses and their practice on a daily basis. They too experience frustrations due to feeling overpowered. A chief nurse administrator in a recent study (Brown, 1987) stated, about her own situation:

*I felt I could do nothing for myself or the nurses under this administration.
I had no power. So, I left my position.*

Both these situations involved nurses' experiences of being overpowered in their work settings. Feeling overpowered is a common experience for those working in the bureaucratic hierarchies of hospitals. Brown's (1987) study of the powering process illuminated the theme of overpowering in relationships among persons working in health care delivery systems. In this study, overpowering emerged as one person imposing his or her will on another, irrespective of the wishes of the other. The other is left with a sense of diminished control and, in some cases, a sense of diminished self. The potential for growth is stifled and growth is essential to health and well being of persons in organizations. Another theme, the other side of the powering process, was empowering. Empowering emerged as sharing control, responsibilities, and rewards among persons at all levels of organizations. Persons experience a sense of fulfillment, knowing that they contribute to the work of the organization in meaningful ways, and that they are respected and valued for their contribution.

Nurse administrators, by virtue of position, often hold the key to power for nurses in health care delivery systems. They also hold the key to the way caring, as the essence of nursing, is lived in health care systems. Nurse administrators who are committed to caring in their practice of nursing administration empower their nursing staff, thus promoting health and growth. How does the nurse administrator demonstrate caring in practice? Brown's (1987) work revealed a difference between authentic caring and caretaking by nurse administrators. Authentic caring, as enacted through empowering in relationships, promotes self-actualization and growth (Mayeroff, 1971) whereas caretaking, as enacted in overpowering relationships, promotes a diminishment of the potential of the human spirit. Here I will explore authentic caring and caretaking as expressed through everyday powering relationships between and among people in health care organizations. Authentic caring lived through empowering one another in nurses' ordinary work settings promotes well being for individuals and organizations. Where ill health due to overpowering has been the norm, authentic caring through consistent patterns of empowering is healing by releasing the creative energies of the human spirit.

CARETAKING

Characteristically, caretaking rather than authentic caring by superiors is encouraged in hierarchical bureaucratic organizational structures. Hospitals are the epitome of organizational hierarchy and patriarchy, both historically and presently (Ashley, 1976; Watson, 1990). Not only are hospital structures hierarchical and bureaucratic, but the highest executive positions are usually held by men who enact more traditional, patriarchal, and authoritarian management styles. In these more patriarchal structures, relationships are typically superior-subordinate, with ultimate authority resting with the superior. The superior is cast into the role of caretaker who is responsible for the well being of the subordinate. Often actions taken to enhance this well being are prescriptive, rather than participative with actions taken *for*, rather than *with*, the other. While the motivation of the superior may be benevolent, intending to promote the well being of the subordinate, the effect of caretaking fosters dependency, rather than self-actualization and growth. In organizational hierarchy, the superior is expected to take the perspective of knowing what is best for subordinates and for the organization. Both superiors and subordinates live the roles expected of them by the organization. The system appears to work well if the superior is benevolent and to disintegrate when the superior is harsh. Yet, in both cases, what occurs is disrespectful of persons. Both the potential for self-management of professional affairs and individual contributions to the organization's well being are diminished.

Caretaking has been defined in the literature on codependency as doing for others what they can, and should be doing for themselves (Schaef, 1986; Beattie, 1987; Schaef & Fassel, 1988). Expressed in caretaking roles, as well, is this central theme: the need to control in order to meet personal needs. Kets de Vries and Miller (1984) identified the tendency, in organizations, for a few top executives to set the tone for the whole organization. They influence the strategies, structures, and cultures of organizations through the influence of their personalities. When such key persons exhibit unhealthy behaviors on a consistent basis, the organization begins to mirror those disorders (Kets de Vries & Miller, 1984; Schaef, 1988). For women, codependent, caretaking behaviors are common. In fact, such behaviors are encouraged by our common culture (Schaef, 1986). At the foundation of caretaking behaviors is lack of trust in and respect for both self and other.

In Brown's (1987) study, the deleterious effects of caretaking behaviors were described by participants. Such behaviors were described from the perspective of nurse administrator as superior and subordinate. For example, in the role of the superior, a nurse administrator related:

I would go to the people who worked for me in the nursing department and say, tell me what you need. Let's see how we can work together on those things, but I never let people think I wasn't going to be in charge and have the final word. And I think that was wrong.

This person realized the controlling behaviors she began with were not the way she now chose to enact her administrative role. She described them as controlling and inhibiting for subordinates. Another nurse administrator described the caretaking nature of some nurse administrators:

> *Very motherly. That's the word that comes to mind. You carry people along, cover for them, hold their hands . . .*

This description comes across as "smothering," inhibiting the growth that occurs through making mistakes and learning from them and from making a full contribution to work of the organization.

Both of these examples describe caretaking behaviors from the perspective of the superior. They are overpowering behaviors that foster dependency, rather than interdependency for participants. Nurse administrators were also the recipients of caretaking behaviors in situations where they were "protected" from doing financial planning and budgeting for their organization and where decisions for their departments were made *for* them, rather than *with* them. In all cases, caretaking was controlling and overpowering resulting in stifled growth.

When considering the way power develops in relationships, a single and exclusive perspective is taken too often. Power is described from the perspective of the superior or the subordinate, but does not take into account the interrelationships of the actors. One concern for upper level nurse administrators was their desire for all nurses to participate actively in the organization and their frustration when they did not. For example, a nurse administrator stated:

> *There are also some nurses who don't like responsibility at all. They really don't want to be accountable. They would rather have a they out there be responsible for something.*

In some cases, nurses seem to invite caretaking responses. Nurses may present problems to nursing administration, and expect that a solution will be found by the superior. The problem may be presented as a complaint, but characteristically, there is no expectation of the presenter being involved in creating a solution. Such situations are common in nursing administration, partly because nurses have grown used to hierarchical bureaucracies, with authority and responsibility for most decisions resting with the superior. Manthey (1990) describes this dependency producing mode of management as "Mama Management." The superior is expected to "take care of" the subordinate.

A nurse administrator described her frustration with the traditional bureaucratic authority system. Her statement summarizes the plight of many nurses working in hospitals and other hierarchical, bureaucratic systems.

I had absolutely no power to accomplish what I thought would be best for patient care, nor for the nurses working on that unit. I think that this is the kind of lack of control, control over our own lives, lack of power, that nurses who are in the work situation, particularly in acute-care hospitals, face all the time. There is always someone who is determining what they are going to do. And then we wonder why nurses are not self-starters. We wonder why they don't do things without being told to do them first, and I think this is why. (Brown, 1987)

Caretaking is part of a constellation of experiences leading to overpowering in relationships. Caretaking inhibits growth for persons and organizations. Persons may engage in caretaking, or may invite caretaking, for satisfaction of unhealthy personal needs or in response to organizational expectations. In any case, caretaking is not authentic caring which fosters the well being and growth of the other (Noddings, 1984; Mayeroff, 1971; Watson, 1979). Conversely, caretaking may result in unhealthy modes of dependence for both individual and organization.

AUTHENTIC CARING

Authentic caring by nurse administrators is expressed, in part, through empowering others in the organization. The essence of caring through empowering involves allowing others to act on behalf of themselves and the organization. The central theme in authentic caring is allowing freedom, freedom to be, become, and to actualize one's self as well as the freedom to exercise self-control over individual actions and being. Promotion of self-actualization, both for self and other, is a further expression of caring through empowering in relationships. Watson (1979) considers self-actualization to be the highest human need. Mayeroff (1971) believes that caring for another means to help that person grow and actualize the self. Authentic caring is empowering of the other and is characterized by trust in and respect for the other. The nurse administrator who expresses authentic caring through empowerment is the nurse administrator who allows co-equality between superiors and subordinates. In being co-equal, the unique contribution of each person in the organization is valued. Persons are expected to work together to seek solutions to mutual problems. For example, a nurse administrator in Brown's (1987) study stated:

> *I consider our nurse administrator team to be an entity. The team kind of administration is very important to me. I told them when I came that I would never have that job by myself. And if they were willing to have the job with me, that was O.K. I would never take that job without the nurses' support.*

For this nurse administrator, each person's contribution, including her own, was both valued and expected.

Another aspect of authentic caring is trusting and valuing competence. Several nurse administrators spoke about belief in the competence of the nursing staff. For example:

> *I really value competency, high levels of intellectual achievement, and doing a good job. No matter what you do, I expect you to do that well, and to like doing that.* (Brown, 1987)

And another spoke about trusting in the competence of the nurses in her department:

> *There is no question about whether they (the nursing staff) are capable of doing that. I know that they are and I just expect competence.* (Brown, 1987)

With trust in the competence of the staff, this nurse administrator could allow greater autonomy and freedom, fostering increased contribution to the work of the organization.

Authentic caring is expressed through empowering others, promoting self-direction, and encouraging ownership of both problems and solutions. Health and well being are fostered, the human spirit is enhanced. Reciprocal growth for persons, organizations, and the nursing profession is nourished. Persons experiencing authentic caring are empowered and describe exhilaration and joy in their work. They know they are important to the organization, and they grow.

WAYS OF CREATING AUTHENTIC CARING
THROUGH EMPOWERMENT

How do caring nurse administrators create empowering situations in their everyday practice? Nurse administrators reported employing several approaches that worked for them. Each of the approaches is grounded in authentic caring expressed through empowering actions that foster mutual growth.

One successful approach was to expect the involvement of the other. This requires trust in the abilities of the other and an expectation that the other desires to contribute to the work of the organization. It also requires clear communication of expectations. Argyris (1981) and McGregor (1981), both classical management theorists, speak to this idea. McGregor (1981) delineates basic assumptions about human nature that underlie ways administrators choose to enact their roles. In Theory Y, persons are assumed to be "basically self-directed and creative at work if properly motivated. Therefore, it should be an essential task of management to unleash this potential in individuals" (Hersey & Blanchard, 1988, pp. 54–55). A belief foundational to this notion is that people have the ability to be self-motivated. Since abilities are not automatically enacted, situations must be created to encourage their actualization. The nurse administrator, through an undergirding philosophy of authentic caring in practice, creates these empowering situations. For example, a nurse administrator reported a strong belief in the abilities of employees, and equally strong expectations of them. These expectations, when enacted, promote self-direction and growth for the persons working for her. She stated:

I try desperately to get that inner value of self-worth, self-being into my staff so that they don't have to feel that there's a they out there making all the decisions for them, or a director of nursing sending down the decisions to them. They have the right, the obligation, and the responsibility to do that, and they will be held accountable for it as well. (Brown, 1987)

Another aspect of authentic caring is being patient and persevering in the bid for participation, to include both identification of problems and the creation of solutions. Rather than expecting the superior to solve problems for subordinates, an overall pattern of expecting mutuality in the creation of solutions prevails. The difference is critical. Nurse administrators who are authentically caring see themselves as facilitators of the actions of others, rather than as controllers of those actions. In facilitating, as control rests with the individual performing the actions, so does accountability. Here nurse administrators see their role as creating opportunities for others to contribute. For example, a nurse administrator reported patiently waiting for a head nurse to take responsibility for solving her own unit problems. She not only created the opportunity, but also consistently insisted that the head nurse act as an autonomous agent. She was able to allow the time and opportunity for growth. When talking with the director of nursing, the head nurse stated:

The first six months that I reported to you were really difficult for me to understand. I would come to you with problems and I'd go away and you didn't solve any of them. It took me six months to figure out that you really wanted me to solve them myself. Once I figured it out, you have been the greatest supervisor I ever had! (Brown, 1987)

The ability to patiently wait for growth, a quality of authentic caring for nurse administrators, involves understanding the world of the other and having faith in the process essential for self-actualization. Authentic caring does not demand perfection in performance or that the person come to the work setting with all competencies fully developed. Authentically caring nurse administrators recognize that the work of self-actualization, of being and becoming through caring, is a lifelong process worthy of respectful patience. They understand that growth occurs at differing rates for different persons and that individuals will continue to grow at different rates throughout life. Another nurse administrator spoke about nurses bringing their problems to her to solve, because that was what had been done prior to her taking on her role as the chief nurse executive. She said:

They (the nurses) would say, what are you going to do about that? And I would say, let's see what we can figure out, or I would let them know that I was sure they could handle the problem. (Brown, 1987)

Part of patiently waiting may be weathering the anger of the other because the nurse administrator is not behaving according to the other's expectations. Nurses accustomed to being taken care of may feel frustrated by any increased expectations inherent in demands for greater participation. One cannot assume, at least initially, that all employees want to take on more responsibility, particularly if they have been socialized into the more passive roles expected in rigid, patriarchal bureaucracies. Communicating a belief in their potential is part of authentic caring.

Allowing others and self to make mistakes and valuing the learning that occurs from such mistakes is another important aspect of the process of expressing authentic caring through empowerment. Yet such allowances do create particular difficulties in nursing. Our history demands perfection; we demand perfection of students, staff, and ourselves. Allowing mistakes involves trusting in the competence of the other, thus encouraging innovation and creativity. Typically, bureaucracies foster only "tried and true" modes of operating. However, the current turbulent and unsettled (Emory & Trist, 1978; Garner, Smith, & Piland, 1990) health care environment demands new ways of seeing situations and creating new ways of responding. Morgan (1986), in his now classic work in organizational theory, speaks of imaging a single organization in numerous ways. The more ways a person sees a situation, the more potential responses will be found. The more persons involved in this activity, the greater the potential for highly creative ideas. In the creation of innovative solutions, the nurse administrator must acknowledge that some ideas, when put into practice, will not work. There will be mistakes. Highlighting this notion, a middle manager in nursing spoke about her superior's trust in her and how she felt free to risk new ways of management in her work:

> *The more confidence she [her superior] has in me, the more I'm going to move, and the more risks I'm going to take. I know I can "screw up," and it isn't going to be the end of the world either. I don't have the fear that I must succeed all of the time and make the right decision all of the time. I know that I'm going to make mistakes sometimes, and I know that she's going to allow me to do that!* (Brown, 1987)

By allowing room for error, the superior in this situation supported maximum creativity and growth for the subordinate. The subordinate was empowered through the authentic caring of the superior.

The process of allowing mistakes also extends from subordinate to superior. The subordinate comes to trust the competence of the superior, but allows for less than perfection. There is an acknowledgment of the essential humanity of one another, to include frailty and imperfection. Thus, freedom to create is fostered through mutual relationships among all parties and new, more efficient and effective ways of providing care for clients may be generated.

Yet another essential ingredient of empowering as an expression of authentic caring is affirmation of the other. Affirming validates the worth of the other to the work of the organization and to the person of the nurse administrator. In affirming, the nurse administrator recognizes the contribution of the other, whether superior or subordinate, to the organization. For example, a nurse administrator made the following statement:

> *I want so desperately for them to know that I do appreciate what it is that they [staff nurses] do. And one way to do that is by being up there and being a little more involved with them, letting them know I appreciate their involvement.* (Brown, 1987)

Mutual affirmation provides the fuel for continued expression of authentic caring through empowering.

In summary, several ways to express authentic caring through empowering relationships have been described: avoiding the invitation for caretaking, being patient and persevering in the invitation for participation, expecting involvement, allowing for mutual decisions, allowing mistakes, and affirming one another.

CONCLUSION

The detrimental effects of overpowering as a dominant pattern of interaction in organizations on the well being of organizations and persons working in organizations are clear. Persons who feel consistently overpowered are at risk for negative health outcomes. At the very least, they do not achieve the high level of energy exchange necessary for creative contributions to the workplace. At the same time, the constructive effects of empowering, as a dominant pattern, are also clear. Empowering is energy enhancing. Empowered persons feel an exuberant sense of well being allowing them to contribute to the organization with minimum inhibition.

By calling the disparity of caretaking and authentic caring roles to consciousness, and reflecting on their meaning in everyday nursing practice, nurses may be more successful in creating empowered practice for self and others. Through empowering, we will heal the ills of overpowering by caretaking and unleash unbounded creative energy.

REFERENCES

Argyris, C. (1981). Interpersonal barriers to decision making. In M. T. Matteson & J. M. Ivancevich (Eds.), *Management classics* (pp. 311–331). Santa Monica, CA: Goodyear Publishing Co.
Ashley, J. A. (1976). *Hospitals, Paternalism, and the Role of the Nurse.* New York: Teacher's College, Columbia University.
Beattie, M. (1987). *Codependent no more.* Center City, MN: Hazelden.
Brown, C. L. (1987). Power and images of nursing in the lived worlds of nurse administrators. *Dissertation Abstracts International, 48* (11), 3247-B.
Emery, F. E., & Trist, E. L. (1978). The causal texture of organizational environments. In J. M. Shafritz & P. H. Whitbeck (Eds.), *Classics of organization theory.* Oak Park, IL: Moore Publishing Co.
Garner, J. F., Smith, H. L., & Piland, N. F. (1990). *Strategic nursing management: Power and responsibility in a new era.* Rockville, MD: Aspen.
Hersey, P., & Blanchard, K. H. (1988). *Management of organizational behavior: Utilizing human resources.* Englewood Cliffs, NJ: Prentice-Hall.

Kets de Vries, M. F. R., & Miller, D. (1984). *The neurotic organization*. San Francisco: Jossey-Bass.

Manthey, M. (1990). From "mama management" to team spirit. *Nursing Management, 21*(1), 20-21.

Mayeroff, M. (1971). *On caring*. New York: Perennial Library, Harper & Row.

McGregor, D. M. (1981). The human side of enterprise. In M. T. Matteson & J. M. Ivancevich (Eds.), *Management classics* (pp. 256-264). Santa Monica, CA: Goodyear Publishing Co.

Morgan, G. (1986). *Images of organization*. Beverly Hills, CA: Sage Publications.

Noddings, N. (1984). *Caring: A feminine approach to ethics & moral education*. Berkeley, CA: University of California Press.

Schaef, A. W. (1986). *Co-dependence: Misunderstood-mistreated*. San Francisco: Harper & Row.

Schaef, A. W., & Fassel, D. (1988). *The addictive organization*. San Francisco: Harper & Row.

Watson, J. (1979). *Nursing: The philosophy and science of caring*. Boston: Little, Brown & Company.

Watson, J. (1990). The moral failure of the patriarchy. *Nursing Outlook, 38*(2), 62-66.

12

Creating an Environment in the Hospital Setting that Supports Caring via a Clinical Practice Model (CPM)

Bonnie Wesorick

This paper goes beyond discussion related to caring. It is about how to create and maintain an environment in the clinical practice arena that not only promotes and holds the nurse accountable for caring services, but also, and more importantly, facilitates, guides, and encourages the development and practice of those caring services unique to nursing. The information shared in this paper is the result of seven years of implementation experience in multiple hospitals using the Wesorick Clinical Practice Model (CPM) designed to achieve that end.

Today the majority of all nurses practice in the hospital setting. The need for this setting to have an environment that *consciously* supports the beliefs and truths of caring is essential. Caring will never be the "essence" of nursing unless it is a norm in this practice arena. The realities of the hospital setting are known by the thousands of nurses who practice in this environment and expressed in the literature by some of our colleagues as follows:

Because of the one-sided perspective of the traditional health care (illness-cure) system, caring values of nurses and nursing have become submerged.

135

Furthermore, the concepts of a human care function of the nurse is threat-ened by the technology, the machine, the high-intensity pace of manage-ment, the administrative tasks, and the manipulation of people acquired to meet the needs of the system. (Watson, 1986)

It may be agreed that the prevailing meaning perspective of many nurses are dominated by either a medical or institutional model. (Rogers, 1989)

In general, the concepts, principles, and practices related to human care have not been institutionalized as a nominative expectation of nursing, and so the chance of care being a major part of nursing education and nursing services cannot be ensured. (Leininger, 1986)

Most nursing care is institutionally based and is a clearly perceived aspect of the professional role. (Brenner et al., 1986)

The realities of the hospital setting and the need to change the environ-ment and support the unique caring services of nurses is not just a realization of the profession, but has been addressed by consumers, health advocates, and philanthropic organizations, as noted below.

- John Naisbitt (1982) noted that consumers today demand that health care "balances the wonder of medical technology with the spiritual demands of human nature."
- Pew Charitable Trusts and the Robert Wood Johnson Foundation (1988) formed a grant program called "Strengthening Hospital Nurs-ing: A Program to Improve Patient Care." These foundations joined together to support programs designed to remove the well-known barriers faced by the bedside nurse who provides the unique caring services of nursing.
- The National Commission on Nursing Implementation Project (NCNIP) (1989) has called for the service setting to create environ-ments supported by delivery systems that "promote the optimal out-come for the consumer while providing a satisfying work experience for the provider."
- The Society of Critical Care Medicine, in the publication *Critical Care State of the Art* (Taylor, 1991), will bring the results of a consen-sus conference, "Fostering More Humane Care—Creating a Healing Environment," that clearly states, "The practice setting typically has not provided the tools and resources for the caregiver which facilitate the provision of humane care to the patients and loved ones."

All nurses face the challenge to create an environment that supports the art and science of caring. Yet there are no quick fixes that lead to this type of environment. It is a process of transformation that requires clarity, commitment, accountability, planning, innovation, and time. To create and then maintain the type of environment conducive to caring also demands diligence and intelligence.

Donabedian (1982) notes that proper system design is the most important means of protecting and promoting quality care. Wesorick (1990) notes that nurses practicing in multiple hospitals across the country have not created or implemented systems within the institutional setting to support the art and science of caring. Existing systems are simply designed to support the medical model of care. Following experience with hospitals throughout the country, this author has found that without a clinical practice model that establishes a framework for the practice setting, the process will be random, segmented, and unsuccessful. The following information provides a brief overview of the Wesorick Clinical Practice Model (CPM) designed to create environments that focus on the caring services of nursing and, to this date, implemented in multiple hospitals. The CPM addresses the following four goals or objectives, each of which will be reviewed in turn.

Objectives of the CPM:

1. Delineate the nursing services that flow from the scope and process of professional nursing and clarify the art and science of caring.

2. Establish a process whereby staff govern their unique practice.

3. Implement clinically adaptable tools/resources that support nursing's professional services.

4. Strengthen each nurse's clarity, commitment, and valuing of professional nursing services and their ability to educate peers, other health care providers, and consumers.

Objective One: Delineate the nursing services that flow from the scope and process of professional nursing and clarify the art and science of caring.

Being able to talk about caring or define caring is not enough. Today's Information Age society consumer expects nurses to articulate what caring by nurses really means to them. Roach (1990) stated that caring is not unique to nursing but notes, "Nursing is the professionalization of the human capacity to care through the acquisition and supplication of knowledge, attitudes, and skills required for nursing's prescribed roles." The profession will not be able to assure consistency of caring services unless nurses practicing in the hospital setting can clearly articulate what their unique services are, and value and deliver them with the same expertise that they deliver medical services.

The first challenge, then, is to transform the theory related to caring into actual services so that: the consumer can understand, value, and know what to expect from nursing service; the practitioners can support and hold each other accountable to the specific professional services; and the core beliefs of the profession can easily be related to the services. Listed below are just those core beliefs as defined by the CPM.

The Core Beliefs of the CPM:

- The nurse is licensed to provide a professional service.
- The nurse is privileged to provide service for a person or significant other, each consisting of an integrated physical, psychological, sociocultural, and spiritual dimension.
- The services that nurses provide should be clearly defined.
- The theoretical scope of practice must be transformed into actual services nurses provide. These services must be clearly defined, named, and articulated by the practitioner.
- Nursing services and physician services are interrelated but different. Both are equally important for health prevention, maintenance, and promotion. Within the framework of the medical model, physician services are focused on diagnosing and treating disease. Within the framework of a nursing practice model, the focus is, as defined by the ANA Social Policy Statement (1980), ". . . the diagnosis and treatment of human response to actual or potential health problems."
- The goal of the medical model is to ward off illness, pain, and death. The goal of nursing is to enter into a relationship with the person that empowers them to heal or care for self. This is not a fixing or controlling relationship.
- The professional services that nurses provide should be determined by the needs of the individuals they service, not by the practice setting or by bureaucratic design. Nurses provide services for people during the whole health and illness continuum. The focus for service is not disease-cure.
- Sufficient resource and proper system design are important means of supporting, protecting, and promoting quality nursing care.
- The system design that supports professional caring must be rooted in the following universal characteristics of quality: dignified and individualized, continuous and coordinated, congruent and mutual, adaptable and flexible, stable and cost effective.
- Nursing process provides a basic framework for service delivery.

PROFESSIONAL SERVICES THAT REFLECT
THE UNIQUE CARING OF NURSING

One of the most significant steps in the establishment of a professional practice environment is clear agreement on and commitment to the services nurses should provide. Actions cannot be taken to create a supportive environment for nurses to provide their unique caring service if there is uncertainty over what the services actually are. To facilitate this process, nursing services must be delineated so as to provide the practitioner, interdisciplinary team, and consumers clarity. Saying we care and not delineating what that means is not sufficient. For the sake of clarity, professional services were placed in three categories—delegated, interdependent, and independent (Wesorick, 1990)—that are explained below.

Delegated Nursing Services

Delegated: Those health care services nurses provide which require a physician's order.

This category addresses those services that are needed by the patient to enhance their health, are delivered by the nurse, but require a doctor's order. Although physicians diagnose and treat the disease, the nurse collaborates with the physician in this process and often is responsible for actually carrying out the physician's orders related to diagnosing and treating the disease. The professional nurse does not carry out an order simply because the physician writes it, but because it is a service that the patient needs at that time. This calls for high level professional nursing judgment and decision making. In the research and development of the CPM, it became very clear to this author that the delegated group of services was well-known by most practitioners. In fact, because of institutional expectations and environmental conditions, delegated was seen as the only important service nurses offered. This resulted in a practice norm called "institutional nursing."

Institutional nursing is "a dependent, task-dominated practice wherein the nurse treats the person only as directed by physician orders, hospital policies, and procedures" (Wesorick, 1990). Because the institution was clear about what they wanted from nurses, "to follow or carry out doctors' orders," nursing practice became centered around the tasks associated with doctor's order. Practice then narrowed to segments such as, "Did you get all the doctor's orders carried out?" If you did, then you were a good nurse. Although nurses know there is much more to nursing than carrying out doctors' orders, the time to carry out other nursing services was not supported. Delegated is not just carrying out the doctor's order, however, but assures the patient that the order will only be carried out if it is appropriate for the individual. Such judgment and decision making on the part of the nurse provides true evidence of professional caring.

Interdependent Nursing Services

Interdependent: Those nursing services related to assessing, monitoring, detecting, and preventing potential physiological complications and problems associated with a specific medical diagnosis/health problem or treatment plan.

This category of service assures consumers that when a nurse enters the room, they can count on the nurse not only knowing what the medical diagnosis, health situation or medical treatment is, but also knowing what physiological complication the patient is at risk for because of their specific health situation. For example, if a person is admitted with an MI, the nurse will know that person is at risk for arrhythmias, CHF, and so on. Interdependent service assures the person that the nurse will assess, monitor, detect, and carry out interventions to prevent all potential physiological complications which that person is at risk for. Interdependent of services is not ordered by the doctor nor is it task driven. Rather, it is driven by the judgement of the professional nurse as he or she decides on a course of action.

Because of the following realities, however, there is need for refinement of interdependent service:

- In a 24-hour period in the hospital, 90 percent of services needed by the person is delivered by the nurse while the physician is only at the bedside for approximately 10 minutes a day.
- Acuity of illness is climbing.
- Hospital stays are shorter.
- Technological demands abound.
- The RN shortage continues.

If interdependent service is not provided, patients are at risk. Caring enough to assure this doesn't happen is critical.

Independent Nursing Services

Independent: Those services nurses provide because the person has a certain human response or nursing diagnosis.

This category assures patients that when a nurse enters the room, he or she will never again be seen as a heart, a lung, a kidney, or as a medical diagnosis— a treatment. Each person will be seen as a unique individual who has a physical, psychological, sociocultural, and spiritual dimension. Each person will be seen as a multidimensional individual who is responding to an actual or potential health situation in a special way. The nurse will diagnose and treat or help that person through his or her unique human response to the situation at hand. Independent service says: yes, nurses assess, monitor, detect, and prevent physiological complications, but they also diagnose and treat the human response. The service of diagnosing and treating the human response is equally as important as diagnosing and treating the disease—one is not more important than the other. For example, assuring that a patient with spinal cord injury and paralysis has physical support is no more important than helping him or her cope with his or her body change. One without the other implies that a person can be divided into parts which are equal to the sum. Health care providers know this is not reality. A person is much more than two lungs, one heart, a brain, and two kidneys.

Independent service is closely associated with why nurses enter the profession in the first place. Nurses want to care for individuals and help make a difference in their health. Although "feeling good about practice" is often associated with providing independent services, it is the weakest most inconsistent delivered group of services in the institutional setting. Nurses who barely have time to pass meds, do medical treatments, and get through report on time have little chance to deliver or mature independent services. Yet, as consumers today demand quality care, it is in independent service that they feel assured they will get quality care.

As noted previously, Naisbitt (1982) perceived that consumers today demand that health care "balances the wonder of medical technology with the spiritual demands of human nature." Nursing diagnosis or diagnosing the human response constitutes that balance precisely. Independent nursing services, the very pivot of that balance, comes into its own here. The caring of nursing associated with independent services goes beyond usual human caring and articulates the art of science or the caring unique to nursing.

Because of the typical environment in the hospital, this component of professional nursing is weaker, less defined, and not as mature as other components. Because nursing's focus on human response has been minimal, nurses themselves often do not value independent services as much as delegated and interdependent services, both of which rely more completely on medical interventions. Developing support systems for a more holistic perspective on caring is essential for the "unique caring of nursing" to become reality. Two specific ways to develop support systems that promote independent nursing services are discussed in objectives two and three that follow.

Objective Two: Establish a process whereby staff govern their practice and care for self.

Joseph (1990) noted that the energetics involved in caring for another can be potentially hazardous to the caregiver. Societal trends coupled with the present technological boom have created physical, ethical, and moral dilemmas that are daily norms for the bedside nurse who enters into a caring relationship with his or her client. Professional hazards that come with caring can be offset, however, if there is a conscious effort and accountability made to create an environment that regenerates or empowers the provider. A term now commonly used in nursing that relates to this type of environment is *shared governance*. The concept of shared governance is one of the critical factors necessary to create an environment that energizes caregivers.

The vision of professional nursing, a vision necessary to create consistencies and norms for caring, and the environment necessary to support professional nursing, is grounded in the implementation of shared governance. This author has had the privilege of listening to many nurses share their visions or hopes for nursing. It isn't that the vision is unclear; it is just that so many struggle as to what their role is in making that vision reality. Shared governance is a valuable key to the actualization of a professional practice environment that empowers practitioners. The implementation of shared governance in multiple settings has revealed the following core beliefs:

- It sees the profession of nursing as a whole with members in practice, education, management, and research tracks.
- It is not track-driven, but track-integrated with joint responsibility for outcome.
- It must be rooted in the core beliefs of the profession of nursing.
- It demands a clear vision from all its members of those services of the profession.
- It is newly named and discussed but is and was a universal desire, a hope that has always been present in the profession.
- It is hard to name but not hard to value.
- It is an innate component of evolving humanity as well as an evolving profession.
- It is not an organizational chart or governmental phenomena.
- It is not participatory, but espouses ownership of the profession by all members of the profession.

- It is an integrated and interactive process that forms the foundation of collegial relationship.
- It is based on the beliefs of human dignity, respect, collaboration, and collegiality of the profession's members.
- It unleashes the power of nursing in each of its members.
- It is not a motionless theory, but a living continuous process.
- It promotes trust, autonomy, choices, alliance, accountability, ownership, integrity, innovation, cohesion, consistency, and congruency.
- It is a process that makes it safe to make mistakes.
- It erases guilt, anxiety, fear, paranoia, control, and powerlessness.
- It is the heartbeat, the fuel, the power needed for a satisfying change or process of transformation.
- It is the process that simply creates empowered professionals.

Nurses cannot engage freely in their own experience if they find themselves in a dualistic, mechanistic, bureaucratic environment typical to hospital settings. Shared governance establishes norms that place professionals in decision-making roles so as to transform the environment to support the provision of excellence in care. In addition, shared governance creates an environment that offers professional diversity and significant choices. In this light, the CPM establishes the process of shared governance via a unit-based practice governance system. Practitioners are empowered to have control and accountability for their practice. When practitioners have the freedom to create an environment that makes it easy for them to give excellent patient care, they do not suffer burn out but become innovative.

Objective Three: Establish a provision for sufficient tools and resources that support the scope and process of practice.

Shifting the powerful bureaucratic environment to support a system designed to enhance professional nursing instead of institutional nursing is hard work. Naisbitt and Aburdene (1985) noted that "the only way to translate vision and alignment into people's day to day behavior is by grounding these lofty concepts in the company's day to day environment." While the concept of caring may not be as lofty, its historic lack of support combined with the presence of many barriers to its fulfillment may make it seem so. However, the tools and resources necessary to support the scope and core beliefs of practice require that, in each step of nursing process, problem solving and critical thinking be developed and integrated into a system driven by the following attributes of quality identified by Donabedian (1987): dignity and individualized, continuous and coordinated, congruent and mutual, adaptable and flexible, stable and cost effective. As a constant reminder of the importance of caring, an integrated process was created in CPM which interfaced the core belief of professional caring into the communication and documentation system used in daily practice.

The tools/resources are: holistic assessment tool, unique plan of care process, interdependent and independent standards of care, outcome-based nurses' notes, professional exchange report process, and significant event and discharge summary format. All tools were interrelated and interactive.

Nursing Profile

The nursing profile is one of the first tools implemented with CPM. In the past, the admission history and physical examination consisted mainly of physiological information, or physiologic history, such as heart sounds, bowel sounds, and lung sounds, with little information on the *person as an individual*. This vital documentation tool—the nursing profile—was altered so as to support the nurse in capturing the person's unique story or capturing their "personhood." The tool was designed to help the nurse connect with the person and see him or her as multidimensional and consisting of a physical, psychological, sociocultural, and spiritual dimension. The tool became a daily visual reminder to all staff of a unified commitment to care for all people as multidimensional individuals. It became a daily visual reminder that the caring services of nursing were different from the physiological caring services of physicians and required a different relationship with different information. Under institutional nursing, the only tools available to the bedside practitioner focused on the medical model of service or physiological story. This tool facilitated the ability of the practitioner to identify strengths as well as the person's concerns in order to potentiate the providers ability to establish mutual goals, prioritize care, maximize person's strengths, and mobilize the person's resources to help them deal with their concerns. (See Addendum A for the admission history component of the profile.)

Standards of Care

The second tool provides the standards of care for the interdependent and independent group of services. (See Addendum B as an example of an Independent Standard [Nursing Diagnosis Categories: Post Trauma Syndrome] and Addendum C as an Interdependent Standard [Care of the Person with Aids]). The standards become a constant reminder to the practitioner that nursing care related to the interdependent and independent services are equally important as those related to the medical model services. The standards were developed and placed in a written format to demonstrate nurses are not task driven or physician order driven, but goal driven, based on desired patient outcomes. The standards provided a common ground for the practitioner and a message of the commitment for these services. The practitioner needed this type of clarity and reinforcement during the transformation process from institutional to professional nursing. Without these tools and a process to integrate them into the nurses daily care and communication/documentation systems, there was no consistency, maturation, or accountability to these unique services.

Plan of Care

Historically, the plan of care was never seen as a valued part of the bedside practitioner's day. Everyone in practice is aware of the blatant failure of the so-called care plan. After intense investigation and now seven years of implementation experience, the nursing care plan (NCP) issue has been clarified. When the concept of NCP is clearly understood, it is very disconcerting to hear that "a nursing care plan is not necessary." While the NCPs of the past are *absolutely* not necessary, the concept of nursing having a plan of care is essential.

The plan of care is an extension of the person's story. That is why it is physically attached to the person's history or overview. It moves into the concept of communicating to other professionals what is important in achieving the mutually desired outcomes of the person nurses are privileged to serve. The purpose of the plan of care is to assure continuity of care by documenting the patient's needs, concerns, problems, and describing personalized approaches to reach desired patient outcomes. This type of mutuality is a continuous process. Mutuality prevents "neutral, biostatic or biocidic" behavior and moves nursing into a "biogenic or bioactive" model of practice as discussed by Halldorsdottir (1990). It clearly demonstrates the caring that is unique to nursing.

An approach to facilitate the plan of care process was developed. When standards of care are available for the practitioner, a plan of care can be written in a time-saving manner. Figure 12-1 exemplifies a plan of care that can be written when standards are available.

Date/Initial	Prob. No.	Re-solved	Needs/Problems Interdependent/Independent	Mutual Goals/Outcome Standards	Nursing Intervention/Process Standards	Altered Dates/Init.
JB 4/10/88	1		Care of the patient with Pneumonia (RLL).	As written	As written. Drinks very little fluids normally – needs reminders – will drink when offered. Likes 7-Up and apple juice "best."	
BT 4/11/88	2		Dysfunctional Grieving related to loss of husband two years ago, no support system, living alone, frequent use of Valium "to treat feelings."	As written. Decrease use of Valium to "treat feelings."	As written. Clarify her use of Valium for grieving and explain its effects. Notified volunteer companion and Widow Support Group.	BT 4/12/88

Figure 12-1
Nursing Care Plan

Standards of care are not to be written out in the plan but are professional expectations of service for which nurses hold each other accountable. Only variance or individualized data is written out. The plan of care is not a place for the nurse to tell another nurse how to practice. It is a place to inform another colleague what is important in the continuous care of one individual.

Documentation and Communication Tools

Tools to support professional documentation and communication associated with the caring services were created. Nurses' notes were developed based on nursing process, functional health patterns, and goal evaluation. Documenting outcomes, based on the person's progress toward mutually set goals, was a major change and brought the concept of caring to another level. An education record designed to document the teaching–learning process in a brief but concise manner was instituted. In addition to documentation, a professional exchange report process was established that centered around the patient's progress towards mutually determined desired outcomes. The professional exchange process was completely different from the process used in institutional nursing which was centered around reporting on what physician's orders were carried out, or how many delegated services were completed. It focused on the unique health care situation which the nurse was mutually addressing with the person. In addition, the results of changing the documentation and reporting process to be centered around the individual's needs and progress decreased the bedside nurse's paper work and reporting time.

Objective Four: Strengthen each nurse's clarity, commitment, and valuing of professional nursing services and each nurse's ability to educate peers, other health care providers, and consumers.

The fourth objective can only be accomplished if there is a commitment and beginning process of implementation for the other three objectives. Before an environment can be created that supports the "art and science of caring," nurses themselves first must be clear as to what professional nursing is about, be confident in their ability to have control and accountability for that practice, and start creating the support system in the environment they need to make it happen. The greatest challenge faced during the implementation of a program designed to create an environment that supports the unique caring of nurses is the *conscious transformation of the individual nurse's beliefs, values, and assumptions of nursing, both personally and as a whole.* The right environment will stimulate nurses to teach each other, be clear on what they stand for, and unite on core issues. As the practitioner creates that type of environment and strengthens personal clarity and commitment to professional services, the education of peers, the consumer and other health care providers will take place. One cannot occur without the other.

CONCLUSION

Today the hospital setting is driven by cost-containment pressures, competitive business issues, informed consumers, complex health needs, aging population, technological mushrooming, and nursing shortage realities. The attempt to transform this historically bureaucratic environment based on the medical model to a place where the unique caring services of nursing can be received by all who seek health care is a massive undertaking. After seven years of such effort with many nurses across the country, we have made inroads but still have much work to do and much to learn from each other. Together we have learned that any program designed to support an environment of caring must be integrated, interactive, and mature the vision of professional nursing. Just having enough staff, *or* offering continued education, *or* making charting easier, *or* having standards of care, *or* using new assessment tools, *or* offering self-scheduling, *or* implementing shared governance *or* having primary or case management will not create an environment that supports caring. A holistic approach is not only essential for excellence in nursing care but also essential in creating an environment that not only supports nurses, but also helps them develop and mature those services associated with caring.

Deming (1987) notes that talking or creating words, slogans, or inspirational words about important things, such as caring, does nothing. He notes, "Beyond the momentary inspiration the words may evoke in us, we need to have a method by which to achieve the promised goal of the message." The method, the work process, by which the goals are to be achieved must accompany the inspirational statement of the goal. That is the purpose and reason for success of the CPM.

The call to be a "compassionate healer" is one faced by all of us. It may be wise for us to start with caring for each other. Remember the majority of our colleagues practice in an environment that daily blocks compassionate healing. Henry David Thoreau has eloquently described the challenge we all face: "It is something to paint a picture or to carve a statue and so to make a few objects beautiful. But it is far more glorious to carve and paint the atmosphere in which we work to affect the quality of the day. This is the highest of the arts." This describes the work of the CPM.

REFERENCES

American Nurses' Association. (1980). *A social policy statement.* Kansas City: The Author.

Benner, P., Boyd, C., Cervantez, T., Marz, M., Buerhaus, P., & Leininger, M. (1986). The care symposium, considerations for nursing administrators. *Journal of Nursing Administration, 16*(1), 25–30.

Byham, W. (1989). *Zapp: The lightning of empowerment.* Pittsburgh: Development Dimensions International Press.

Deming, E. (1987). *Deming theory of management.* Virginia: Expert knowledge systems, Inc.

Donabedian, A. (1982). *The criteria and standards of quality.* Ann Arbor: Health Administration Press.

Ferguson, M. (1980). *The aquarian conspiracy.* Los Angeles: J.P. Tarcher, Inc.

Halldorsdottir, S. (1990). *Four basic modes of being with another.* Twelfth International Caring Conference, Houston, Texas.

Joseph, L. (1990). *The energetics of conscious caring for the compassionate healer.* Twelfth International Caring Conference, Houston, Texas.

Leininger, M. (1986, July). *Care facilitation and resistance factors in the culture of nursing Topics in clinical nursing,* 7–12.

Naisbitt, J. (1982). *Megatrends.* New York: Warner Books.

Naisbitt, J., & Aburdene, P. (1985). *Reinventing the corporation.* New York: Warner Books.

Naisbitt, J., & Aburdene, P. (1990). *Megatrend 2000.* New York: William Marrow.

PEW Charitable Trusts and Robert Wood Johnson Foundations. (1988). *Strengthening hospital nursing: A program to improve patient care.* Florida: The Author.

Roach, S. (1990). *A call to consciousness: Compassion in today's health world.* Twelfth International Caring Conference, Houston, Texas.

Rogers, M. (1989). Creating a climate for the implementation of nursing conceptual framework. *Journal of Continuing Education in Nursing, 20*(3), 112–116.

Taylor, R. (Ed.) (1991). *Critical care-state of the art.* California: Fullerton.

Watson, J. (1986). *Nursing: Human science and human care, a theory of nursing.* Norwalk, CT: Appleton-Century-Crofts.

W. K. Kellogg Foundation. (1989). *Nursing's vital signs, shaping the profession for the 1990's.* A design for Nursing's Future from the National Commission on Nursing Implementation Project. Michigan: The Author.

Wesorick, B. (1990). *Caring: A service not a slogan.* Proceedings of the Seventeenth Annual National Teaching Institute, California: American Association of Critical Care Nurse.

Wesorick, B. (1990). *Standards of nursing care: A model for clinical practice.* Philadelphia: J.B. Lippincott Co.

ADDENDUM A

BUTTERWORTH HOSPITAL NURSING PROFILE

HISTORY

GENERAL INFORMATION ★

Admission Date / Time _____   Valuables _____   Disposition _____   How to be addressed _____   Status   M   S   W   D

Age _____ Admission Ht: _____ Wt: _____   Emergency contact: Name, Address, Phone _____

T _____ BP _____ P _____ R _____   Next of kin, legal guardian _____

Source of Information / Reliability _____   Temporary family living arrangements _____

HEALTH AND ILLNESS PERCEPTION ★   **STRENGTH** N P/S   **CONCERN** N P/S

★ Reason for this admission as stated by patient / Chief Complaint: _____

_____

Expected length of hospitalization _____   Describe previous general health: (1P-5E) _____

How do you heal (fast-slow)? / What helps you heal faster? _____

★ HEALTH PROBLEMS: adult, childhood: (include time frame / dates)

Medical / Psychiatric _____   Surgeries, Accidents, Injuries, Fractures _____

★ Family Hx? (circle) — Diabetes Cancer Hypertension Cardiac Renal Arthritis TB Allergies Stroke Seizures Anemia

Other: _____

★ Tobacco: Pk / day / yr. _____   Caffeine: _____

★ Alcohol _____   Street / Recreational drugs: _____

Substance Abuse Rehab _____

★ **Medication Schedule (Prescription — non-prescription)**

Medication	Dose	Times / Circle last dose	Medication	Dose	Times / Circle last dose

Any medications brought into hospital?   Yes   No   If yes, disposition _____

Is there anything that interferes with your ability to follow health advice or your medication schedule? _____

★ ALLERGIES (Drugs, Anesthesia, Foods, Soaps, Others) _____   Describe Reactions _____

COGNITIVE & PERCEPTUAL: **STRENGTH** N P/S   **CONCERN** N P/S

★ Vision Problems: nearsighted   farsighted   stigmatism   blurring   tearing   diplopia   cataracts   glaucoma

surgeries   pupil asymmetry _____   ★ aids (glasses, contacts R/L, implant) _____

Problems reading? _____

Hearing: (★ aids R L) _____   ★ Communication: aphasic, dysphasic, language barrier _____

★ Pain Experience: describe pain threshold / tolerance on a scale of 1-5 _____

★ How do you respond to pain? _____

★ What makes your pain better / worse? _____

★ Thought Process: describe changes in memory (recent / remote), learning abilities, decision-making _____

★ What methods help you learn (reading, demonstration, group, T.V. pictures) _____

SLEEP-RELAXATION   **STRENGTH** N P/S   **CONCERN** N P/S

★ Sleep times: _____   naps _____

★ Problems: getting to sleep / waking early, recurrent dreams, nightmares, narcolepsy _____

★ Aids / rituals: _____

What helps you to relax? (people / place / things / techniques) _____

ACTIVITY-EXERCISE-SELF CARE   **STRENGTH** N P/S   **CONCERN** N P/S

Usual BP _____   Life style alterations / self care adaptations / equipment / safety considerations

★ **CARDIAC:** circle chest pain, SOB, palpitations, murmurs, fainting, vertigo. Orthopnea, dizziness, pacemaker, nocturnal dyspnea.

★ **PULMONARY:** circle: Hemoptysis, sputum, SOB / DOE, wheezing, coughing, asthma, P.E., recent URI, TB.

★ **PERIPHERAL VASCULAR:** circle varicosities, edema, claudication, vascular access: Hickman, Portacath, etc. bleeding disorders, D.V.T.

★ **NEURO-MUSCULAR-ORTHO:** circle seizures, cramps, spasms, discomfort, stiffness, altered sensation, numbness / tingling, decreased ROM, muscular weakness

★ **IMMUNE:** steroids, Infections (acute / chronic), HIV / AIDS, Hepatitis

What do you do to keep healthy? Exercise pattern (work, recreational) _____

What activities are most important to you? (hobbies, family, social) _____

Describe energy level (1P-5E) _____ usual _____

★ Grade ADL by 0 = independent, 1 = needs equipment, 2 = needs equipment & person, 3 = equipment person, 4 = dependent
Feeding _____ Bathing _____ Dressing _____ Ambulating _____ Toileting _____
Dominant hand L R Aids circle those brought to hospital _____

NUTRITIONAL-METABOLIC | STRENGTH N P/S | CONCERN N P/S

★ Diet / eating habits (restrictions, supplement) _____

Adherence _____ Eating habits good for health? _____
Appetite (1P-5E) Usual _____ Current _____ Who prepares meals _____
Usual Wgt. _____ Time frame for any weight gain / loss? _____
★ Problems: circle — abdominal pain nausea vomiting anorexia bulimia altered taste _____

★ SKIN circle — infections itching moles birthmarks fungus rash lesions bruises dry/oily jaundice edema _____
incisions changes in hair, nails _____

Hygiene pattern _____
★ TEETH Dentures upper _____ lower _____ partial plate _____ proper fit of dentures? yes _____ no _____
Teeth status _____

ELIMINATION | STRENGTH N P/S | CONCERN N P/S

Pattern _____ stool characteristics: _____ ★ last BM: _____
★ GI problems: circle — constipation diarrhea hemorrhoids bleeding incontinence _____
Life style changes _____

★ GU problems: circle — dribbling retention pain urgency frequency hesitancy nocturia discharge sugar hematuria
recent UTI incontinence _____
Lifestyle changes? _____

SELF PERCEPTION | STRENGTH N P/S | CONCERN N P/S

Describe yourself (personality, disposition, mood swings, body image) _____

What makes you 'feel good about yourself? (Self-esteem / self-worth) _____

SEXUALITY-REPRODUCTIVE | STRENGTH N P/S | CONCERN N P/S

Menstruation _____ Last period: _____
★ Problems _____ Pap smear _____
Breast self exam _____ Mammogram _____
Testicular self check _____ Contraceptives: _____
★ History circle — menopause complications with pregnancy douching hot flashes breast tenderness dimpling
nipple changes impotence S.T.D. _____
Do you think this illness may affect your sexuality (expression, femininity, masculinity? Concerns? _____

COPING-INDEPENDENCE | STRENGTH N P/S | CONCERN N P/S

★ List significant losses, major life changes, or stressors in life — note time (divorce, death, job change/retirement, victim of traumatic event.) _____

★ Impact on life _____

How do you cope with loss / stress / change? _____

How can we help you maintain your independence / control? _____

VALUES-BELIEFS | STRENGTH N P/S | CONCERN N P/S

Will this hospitalization affect your plans (goals and dreams)? _____
★ What spiritual, cultural practices / values are important for us to know _____

Support affiliation / spiritual support _____
Would you like to have these affiliations notified? Yes No Done /Date _____

GROWTH AND DEVELOPMENT / ROLE RELATIONSHIPS | STRENGTH N P/S | CONCERN N P/S

Occupation /Retired _____
Living with _____ Children / ages / dependents _____

Family / significant other data (describe relationships, knowledge of / response to illness) _____

Who is able to help you at home? _____
Are there people who depend on you? _____ Who? _____
Housing arrangements / layout (stairs, multi-level) _____
Do you expect to return there? Yes No Where? _____
Anticipate changes because of this illness (job, family, housing) _____

Community services used recently _____
Services anticipated upon discharge _____

Financial concerns: _____
★ What questions, fears or concerns do you have about your health? _____

★ What information (activities, routines, habits) would help us give you more personalized care? _____

BUTTERWORTH HOSPITAL—NURSING STANDARDS

NURSING DIAGNOSIS: *POST TRAUMA RESPONSE (PTR)*

DEFINITION: The state of an individual experiencing a sustained painful response to a traumatic event (situation beyond ordinary experience involving a realistic danger of psychological or physiological destruction which could mobilize fear of death).

RELATED/RISK FACTORS

PERSONAL
Individual constitution:
   age
   sex
   personality
   race
   educational level
Social, cultural, ethnic, religious orientation
Moral, ethical and ideological views
Support system
Educational and vocational status
Level of psychosocial development
Level of coping and problem solving skills
History of unresolved PTR

ENVIRONMENTAL
Actual/perceived traumatic event:
   disaster
   war
   epidemic
   accident
   rape
   assault
   torture

PHYSIOLOGICAL
Health status

TREATMENT RELATED
Actual/perceived traumatic:
   surgery
   illness
   treatment

FACTORS INFLUENCING PTR PROCESS

Pre-existing Condition
Related/Risk Factors

Severity of Trauma
*Intensity, frequency and duration of traumatic events
*Meaning and perception of the trauma

No visible PTR → PTR

Post trauma stressors
   *Personal
   *Environmental
   *Physiological
   *Treatment related

Support Resources

No PTR → PTR

DEFINING CHARACTERISTICS

Note: These represent characteristics that were not present in the individual prior to the traumatic experience.

General Pattern of PTR Resolution

```
                    ┌──────────────────────┐
                    │   TRAUMATIC EVENT    │
                    └──────────────────────┘
                               │
                    EMERGENCY/OUTCRY PHASE
                  Coping goal: Survival & Functioning
                               │
              ┌────────────────┴────────────────┐
              ▼                                  ▼
   ┌────────────────────┐           ┌──────────────────────────┐
   │   INTRUSIVE PHASE  │           │      DENIAL PHASE         │
   │  Coping goal:      │ fluctuation│   Coping goal:           │
   │  Acknowledgement   │◄─────────►│  Reduction of emotional   │
   │  of the traumatic  │           │  impact                   │
   │  events.           │           │                           │
   └────────────────────┘           └──────────────────────────┘
                               │
                               ▼
        ┌───────────────────────────────────────────────────┐
        │            REFLECTIVE/TRANSITION PHASE             │
        │   Coping Goal:                                     │
        │   Development of a realistic view of the traumatic │
        │   events and the aftermath.                        │
        │   Strengthening of the personality traits through  │
        │   grief work.                                      │
        └───────────────────────────────────────────────────┘
                               │
                               ▼
        ┌───────────────────────────────────────────────────┐
        │          COMPLETION/INTEGRATION PHASE              │
        │   Coping goal:                                     │
        │   Integration of the traumatic events into new     │
        │   ego-synthesis.                                   │
        └───────────────────────────────────────────────────┘
```

MAJOR

Re-experience of the traumatic event which may be identified in cognitive, affective, or sensory motor activities.
Flashbacks
Intrusive thoughts
Repetitive dreams, nightmares
Excessive verbalization of traumatic event
Verbalization of survival guilt or about behavior required for survival.

MINOR

Psychic/emotional numbing:
Impaired interpretation of reality
Confusion
Dissociation or amnesia
Vagueness about traumatic event
Constricted affect
Impaired memory
Verbalization of feeling numb, detached, or alienated

Altered life style:
Self-destructiveness
Substance abuse
Suicide attempt
Acting out behavior
Thrill seeking activities that recreate the traumatic event
Difficulty with interpersonal relationships
Social withdrawal, social isolation
Development of phobia regarding trauma
Poor impulse control (irritability, explosiveness)
Emotional lability
Sleep disturbances
Multiple physiologic symptoms (i.e., pains, fatigue, GI disturbances, etc.)
Marked decrease interest in activities
Hyperalertness or exaggerated startle responses
Trouble with memory and concentration
Personality change
Inability to discuss traumatic event
Negative self concept
Loss of faith, existential malaise or meaninglessness

© Used with permission: Wesorick. B.. *Standards of Nursing Care: A Model for Clinical Practice,* J. B. Lippincott, 1990.

153

GOALS/OUTCOME STANDARDS

HEALTH/ACTIVITY

Maintain, reverse, prevent, and or control.
  Defining characteristics.
  Related risk factors.

Measurable criteria for consideration.

1. Verbalize thoughts, feelings and needs, especially those related to the traumatic event.
2. Maintain relationship(s) with significant other(s). (i.e., initiate phone visits with friends and personal visits with close friends.)
3. Identify the cause of anxiety, anger, depression, and loss of control.
4. Identify and utilize effective coping techniques. Control/channel energy, anxiety, anger and depression to appropriate activity.
5. Report adequate rest/sleep for sufficient energy.
6. Develop realistic short-term goals and future plans.
7. Maintain safety without evidence of injury or violence.
8. Discuss impact of the integration of the traumatic event experience into their life.

KNOWLEDGE

Patient/significant others will have knowledge related to Post Trauma Response as evidenced by:

  Verbalization of related/risk factors and defining characteristics.

  Measurable criteria for consideration:
    Express readiness for learning.
    State how related/risk factors and defining characteristics may be modified.
    Demonstrate knowledge and comprehension of teaching.

1. Verbalize that progression through the "General Pattern of PTR Resolution" is a normal and healthy response to the experience of a traumatic event.
2. Identify and make connections with support persons and resources.

State appropriate resources for support.

Individualized measurable criteria to be placed on NCP.

NURSING INTERVENTIONS/PROCESS STANDARDS

HEALTH/ACTIVITY

Assess, monitor and document the defining characteristics and the related/risk factors.

Plan mutually developed goals. Document.

Implement appropriate suggested nursing interventions as follows and document:

1. Establish a trusting, therapeutic relationship by accepting the patient at her/his current level of functioning and by assuming a positive, consistent and nonjudgemental attitude. (Do not view the patient as a villain or victim.)
2. Help the patient talk about the traumatic event.
3. Actively listen in an empathetic, accepting manner to the patient talk about the trauma and its impact on her/him.
4. Discuss why patient may be vulnerable to Post Trauma Response by sharing the "Factors Influencing Post Trauma Response Process."
5. Share your own struggle for meaning and the feelings that are aroused by hearing the patient's story, as appropriate.
6. Assist the patient to plan daily activities as possible and to maintain a balance between solitude and socialization.
7. Help the patient to recognize the possible fear of intimacy which derives from a sense of loss.
8. Assist the patient to identify/utilize/accept support from others.
9. Assist the patient in practicing social skills and assertive communications skills (i.e., role play, act as an example, give feedback, etc.), as appropriate.
10. Arrange for telephone/personal visits with significant other, as appropriate.

11. Instruct family about the importance of frequent, short visits from family members and close friends.
12. Allow for privacy during interactions, as appropriate.
13. Encourage family to discuss the trauma in response to the patient's requests for information.
14. Request family members to bring meaningful personal items for the patient's use.
15. Ask family members to prepare a list of telephone numbers of family/friends for easy patient access.
16. Assess the worries and concerns related to the patient's outside obligations and intervene as appropriate.
17. Stay with the patient and offer support during episodes of high anxiety, as appropriate.
18. Help ventilate, in realistic terms, feelings associated with the traumatic event and to become aware of the link between anxiety/anger/depression and grieving.
19. Encourage patient to identify situations in which they feel anxious, angry, and lose control.
20. Assist patient in identifying and utilizing constructive/socially acceptable ways of expressing energy and anger.
21. Teach relaxation, guided imagery, use of music and other stress reduction techniques of interest to the patient as an effective coping method.
22. Help the patient to think through patterns of feeling, thinking and acting, and assess the benefits/consequences on overall health status.
23. Help the patient to realistically evaluate strengths and weaknesses.
24. Assist patient with setting small goals leading to a self-defined, realistic outcome (so as to increase probability of success).
25. Praise patient for gains in managing ADL's, as appropriate.
26. Set limits for violent/acting out behaviors, as appropriate.
27. Assess the level of violent behavior or suicide risk and take appropriate action.
28. Assist to recognize the effects and consequences of addictions (anything used in excess to control emotional pain, i.e. substance abuse, exercise, work, food) that may lead to psychic numbing, inhibition of grieving, postponed anxiety, increasing health problems.
29. Consult Psychosocial CNS.

Add individualized interventions specific to the patient in the nursing care plan.

Evaluate and document, in nurses' notes, progress toward outcome standards.

KNOWLEDGE

> Assess and document:
>> Readiness to learn.
>> Patient's knowledge/skill level rolated to related/risk factors and defining characteristics.
>
> Plan and document mutually developed goals.
>
> Implement and document
>> Teaching plan to increase knowledge (the specific protocol for related/risk factors, if available) by listing nursing interventions related to:
>>> Steps in learning.
>>> Strategies.
>>> Equipment.
>>> Instruct and/or discuss with patient each factor listed under knowledge outcome standards.
>>> Reinforcement.
>> Confere with consultant(s) as appropriate and document:
>
> (Medical social worker, hospital chaplain, priest, rabbi, or patient's minister, Psychosocial/Unit CNS, patient educators, volunteer companion, social services reference book, child/life specialist, etc.)
>
> Evaluate and document progress toward outcome standards:
> • Modify teaching plan, if appropriate.
> • Refer to appropriate resources, if unable to meet goals by discharge.

BUTTERWORTH HOSPITAL   Authors: Nancy Agents, RN, BSN

Candy Humes, RN, BSN

Julie Chamberlain, RN, MHS, CIC

ADDENDUM C

INTERDEPENDENT STANDARD: CARE OF THE PATIENT WITH ACQUIRED IMMUNODEFICIENCY SYNDROME

GOALS/OUTCOME STANDARDS

By Discharge:
- Person will exhibit no/minimal or control of signs and symptoms of listed potential physiological problems.
- Person/significant other will verbalize an understanding of Acquired Immunodeficiency Syndrome (AIDS) and its impact on lifestyle/present health status.
1. Verbalize the signs and symptoms of AIDS.
2. State how the disease is transmitted.
3. Verbalize why they are at risk for infection.
4. State the name, purpose, dosage, scheduling, major side effects, and the importance of taking medications.
5. State the signs and symptoms of common potential complications and the appropriate action to be taken.
6. State appropriate resources for support (Community AIDS Task Force, Hospice, Wellness Network, AIDS Hot Line).
7. Integrate basic hygienic practices into ADL.

NURSING INTERVENTIONS/PROCESS STANDARDS

Assess, Monitor, and Detect:
- The impact of other pre-existing health problems.
- The impact of diagnostic studies, including lab values (WBC's, HIV Ab, Th/Ts ratio, VDRL, HBsAg, anti HBC, SGOT, SGPT, Hgb, Hct, PTT, ABG's, blood cultures).
- Baseline vital signs and trends.

Assess, Monitor, Detect, and Prevent:
- The following potential problems and implement nursing interventions are appropriate:
INFECTIONS AEB (as evidenced by):
- ↑TPR, early—↑WBC/late—↓WBC; warmth, redness, swelling, drainage, pus, odor, pain, chills, weakness, malaise, (+) cultures, Δ in secretions (consistency, color, odor), fatigue, myalgias, arthralgias, night sweats, Δ in mental status, headache (H/A), nuchal rigidity, backache, photophobia, diarrhea.
- Sepsis: Hemodynamic instability, Δ in B/P, P, RR, wedge pressure, cardiac output, and systemic vascular resistance.
1. Carry out and discuss proper hygiene measures.
2. Carry out and discuss care from principles of clean to dirty.
3. Discuss how to prevent skin irritation/breakdown and correlate to life style pattern, i.e., gardening, avoid temperature extremes, harsh soaps.
4. Discuss the importance of nutrition to prevent infection/promote health; evaluate and support nutrient and fluid intake for basic four; explain the need for protein and calories.
5. Establish a balance between appropriate exercise and rest.
6. Discuss precautions concerning exposure to communicable diseases: avoid crowds, sick children and adults, or children recently vaccinated. Wash hands after contact with pets.

7. Discuss signs and symptoms of infection.
8. Obtain cultures of drainage and/or excretions as appropriate.
9. Utilize cooling measures as appropriate (sponging, hypothermia blanket).

PNEUMONIA AEB:
- Hypoxemia, ↑SOB, ↑TPR, abnormal ABG's, Δ in sputum, Δ in CXR, (+) cultures, cyanosis, diaphoresis, restlessness, tachypnea, dyspnea.
- Pneumocystis carinii (PCP)—same plus ↑ frothy sputum.

TUBERCULOSIS AEB:
- Δ in chest x-ray, ↑TPR, night sweats, weight loss, bloodtinged sputum.
10. Collect sputum for acid fast bacillus smear and culture.
11. Place in respiratory isolation.

HYPOXEMIA AEB:
- ↓pO$_2$, ↑pCO$_2$, ↓O$_2$ sat, ↑P, ↑RR, ↑resp. effort, restlessness, anxiety, diaphoresis, cyanosis, fatigue, Δ in lung sounds, weakness, Δ in mental status.
- Adult Respiratory Distress Syndrome (ARDS) AEB: Severe dyspnea, ↓pO$_2$ despite ↑FiO$_2$, cyanosis, Δ in chest x-ray → (diffuse bilateral infiltration), ↓ or ∅ breath sounds.
- Pneumothorax/hemothorax AEB: ↓ or ∅ BS, plugged CT→ ↓ or ∅ drainage, increasing crepitus, (+) chest x-ray.
12. Suction as appropriate.
13. Facilitate effective C & DB, use of incentive spirometer, early ambulation and position change as appropriate.
14. Assess need for O$_2$ and respiratory therapy.
15. Space ADL's with planned rest periods.

LESIONS AEB:
- Kaposi's Sarcoma—purple/red nodules.
- Viral and fungal lesions → frequent genital and perianal ulcers, oral ulcers or rashes.
16. Demonstrate and discuss good handwashing and cleanliness in daily living practices.
17. Provide comfort measures prn; avoid restrictive clothing, establish turning schedule.
18. Use universal precautions for contact with any blood/body fluids and discuss rationale with patient/significant other.
19. Keep oral membranes moist at all times; offer oral hygiene before and after each meal & at bedtime, use toothbrush, waterpic, sponge toothettes as appropriate.
20. Modify diet i.e., bland, soft, liquid, ↑ calorie & protein, frequent small feedings, avoid citric acid (orange, lemon, tomatoes), excessive hot or cold foods.

GASTROINTESTINAL DISTRESS AEB:
- Diarrhea (acute/chronic), weight loss, dehydration, nausea, vomiting, ↓ Hgb and Hct, ↓ skin turgor, anorexia, ketones in urine, oral or esophageal ulcers.
- HIV wasting syndrome (malnutrition) AEB: weight loss > 10% body weight, diarrhea ≥ 30 days, fever (no known origin) ≥ 30 days with chronic weakness.
21. Monitor cumulative I & O (hour, shift, day) and correlate nutritional intake, caloric counts and weight.
22. Provide a calm, well ventilated, aseptic environment.
23. Discuss approach to use when experiencing nausea (taste bud Δ's, early satiety, nausea from smells, sore mouth).
24. Encourage liquids and offer small frequent meals (↓ residue, ↑ calorie, ↑ protein).
25. Modify diet to ↓ hot & spicy foods, offer cool, bland foods.
26. Institute comfort measures when vomiting subsides (mouth care, allow rest, wash face, offer diversion).
27. Plan with patient for control of bowel incontinence (accessible bathroom facilities, commode, bed pan).
28 Assess for & prevent skin breakdown, perianal cleansing & hygiene after defecation (hand washing, sitz baths, washcloth, etc.).
29. Record number, consistency, and color of stools and note presence of blood.

HIV ENCEPHALOPATHY AEB:
- Confusion, Δ in mental status, uncooperative, refusal to talk, sleep disturbances, delusions, suicidal feelings, dementia, apathy, restlessness, seizures.
30. Provide safe environment.

PAIN AEB:
- Arthralgia, neuralgia, verbalization, restlessness, anxiety, diaphoresis, Δ in vital signs, ↓ eye contact, ↓ attention span, inability to sleep, reluctance to Δ position.
31. Discuss multifaceted origins of pain and mutually establish pain control plan.

KNOWLEDGE DEFICIT
- Refer to the Independent Standard "Knowledge Deficit."
- Instruct and/or discuss factors listed under expected outcomes/goals.
- Identify and individualize the teaching interventions related to AIDS.
32. Collaborate with dietitian and medical social worker regarding discharge planning and AIDS networking resources.
33. Psychosocial nurse to assist patient with coping with illness.
- Evaluate effectiveness of teaching interventions related to AIDS.
- Document and notify physician of significant changes in patient's status and/or presence of signs and symptoms of potential problems.
- Add individualized information that gives direction to nursing interventions, and place on NCP prn.
- Determine the nursing diagnosis category which describes the human response to illness and individualize on NCP.

GENERAL INFORMATION: ACQUIRED IMMUNODEFICIENCY SYNDROME

A. Stages of Illness
   1. *HIV Infection:* Human Immunodeficiency Virus
      a. Virus enters bloodstream → antibody (Ab) produced.
      b. HIV Ab blood test detects presence of Ab, usually two weeks to three months after infection, but can take much longer to develop. Once infected, the person may remain well, but transmits the virus and may infect others, even though his/her Ab is still negative.
      c. When the virus enters the bloodstream, it attacks certain white blood cells (T-lymphocytes) which function to fight infection and are part of the immune system.
      d. The virus is a retrovirus which has a special enzyme (reverse transcriptase). This is a unique enzyme which incorporates the viral DNA into the genetic material of the T-lymphocyte → destruction of that cell → severely weakening the immune system.
   2. *ARC*—AIDS Related Complex:
      a. A pre-AIDS diagnosis that lacks certain diagnostic criteria but may progress to AIDS.
      b. The victim's blood does test positive for the HIV Ab and the virus is present in the blood stream. At this point the victim can infect others with the virus.
      c. An ARC patient does have non-specific signs and symptoms of infection but lacks the opportunistic infections and disease present in patients with AIDS.
   3. *AIDS*—Acquired Immunodeficiency Syndrome:
      a. It is the terminal stage of a viral disease including a variety of specific opportunistic infections and malignancies.
      b. Bacteria, protozoa, fungi, other viruses and malignancies that ordinarily would not survive or develop, now become pathogenic and cause "opportunistic disease" using the opportunity of lowered resistance to infect and destroy.
B. *Nonspecific* signs and symptoms of infection in patients with *ARC* are:
   1. Lymphadenopathy ≥ 2 non-inguinal sites.
   2. Profound, involuntary weight loss, > 10 percent of baseline body weight.

3. Fever ≥ 38 degrees C, intermittent or continuous.
4. Diarrhea lasting > 30 days.
5. Fatigue, malaise and arthralgias.
6. Night sweats.
7. Two or more abnormal laboratory values (↓ T helper cells, anemia, leukopenia, thrombocytopenia etc.).

C. AIDS: These patients have the signs and symptoms of ARC plus one or more of the following diseases or system alterations:

1. *Kaposi's Sarcoma:* Four stages - I. *Cutaneous, local indolent;* II. *Cutaneous, locally aggressive,* ± *regional nodes;* III. *Generalized muco-cutaneous,* ± *nodes;* IV. *Visceral.* Kaposi's Sarcoma is a malignant growth appearing as a reddish purple skin nodule which can occur on any site of the body (trunk, extremities, hard palate, conjunctiva); confirmed by skin biopsy. (Mycobacterium avium intracellulare may be involved). It affects about 34 percent of patients with AIDS, persons are < 60 years of age.

2. Lesions:
   a. Herpes simplex—mucocutaneous lesions on the genitalia, anal or oral tissues persisting > 1 month.
   b. Herpes zoster—disseminated shingles (vescicular lesions) on any skin surface.
   c. Fungus—cryptococcosis may be a pulmonary infiltrate, meningitis, or a fungemia; candidiasis (often nodular lesions) is also found ulcerating in the esophagus, trachea or lungs or develops into a fungemia.

3. *Lymph Nodes:* Lymphadenopathy variable with respect to size, consistency and frequency in patients, prominent in cervical, occipital, axillary and inguinal areas, enlarged spleen in later stages of AIDS. Mycobacterium avium intracellulare may be involved.

4. *Gastroenteritis:*
   a. Anorexia, nausea and vomiting, dehydration (HIV wasting syndrome).
   b. Upper tract—candida infections (oral thrush) or herpetic lesions with dysphagia.
   c. Lower tract—watery diarrhea with many protozoan infections including amebiasis and cryptosporidiosis, bacterial infections such as salmonella; rectal and anal pain with herpes proctitis or invasive perineal herpes.
   d. Cytomegalovirus (CMV) has been isolated from ulcerative gastrointestinal lesions.

5. *Respiratory:*
   a. Non-productive cough, dyspnea at rest or with exertion, abnormal chest x-ray (infiltrates, pneumothorax).
   b. ARDS—Adult respiratory distress syndrome may develop which may lead to mechanical ventilation.
   c. PCP—Pneumocystis carinii pneumonia is the most common respiratory infection. Diagnosed by a lung biopsy via a bronchoscopy. Over 60 percent of patients present initially with this infection. Mortality is about 60 percent per episode of PCP infection.
   d. TB—Mycobacterium tuberculosis is characterized by a productive cough and blood tinged sputum.
   e. Bacterial infections are also frequent.

6. *Central Nervous System:*
   a. Dementia, apathy, psychomotor retardation, acute Guillain-Barré like syndrome with rapid onset of motor weakness. Central Spinal Fluid shows non-specific abnormalities in 60 percent of affected patients.
   b. Cryptococcal meningitis—confusion, chronic low grade headache without nuchal rigidity.
   c. Toxoplasmosis meningitis—confusion, headache, seizure, paresis, nuchal rigidity.

    d. Cytomegalovirus (CMV) often causes encephalitis, confusion, lethargy,
        headaches, etc.
    e. Lymphomas—primary of the brain or non-Hodgkin's lymphoma.
    f. Progressive multifocal leukoencephalopathy.
  7. *Eyes:* Cytomegalovirus (CMV) retinitis. Fundoscopic exam reveals cotton wool
      spots and/or retinal hemorrhages → blindness.
D. Psychosocial
  1. Anxiety, anger, depression, fear are some of the stages of anticipatory grief this
      patient will experience.
  2. Concerns about self-image changes, alienation by family, being totally dependent,
      sexual issues (health of partners, precautions).
  3. Legal and financial questions.
  4. Concerns about community resources and support services.
E. Laboratory Data
  1. HIV antibody blood test (Elisa) repeated and confirmed by positive Western Blot
      test.
  2. Leukopenic (WBC ↓ 3500/mm3), lymphopenic (↓ 1500/mm3).
  3. Liver enzymes, SGOT, SGPT elevated in active or chronic Hepatitis B (common in
      homosexuals and IV drug abusers) presence of Hepatitis B surface antigen
      (HBsAg) and Hepatitis core antibody (anti-HBC).
  4. T-lymphocyte helper (Th) and suppressor (Ts) markers for AIDS and pre-AIDS
      (persistence of a low Th number over a period of 3–6 months).
  5. Positive antibody for Toxoplasmosis (baseline measurement if a patient develops
      CNS symptoms).
  6. Chest x-ray (Pneumocystis carinii pneumonia or T.B.).
  7. Arterial blood gases ($\downarrow O_2$)—metabolic acidosis.
  8. Thromobocytopenia (platelets)—prolonged PT/PTT.
  9. Hemoglobin and hematocrit.
  10. Blood cultures.
F. Routes of Transmission
1. Intercourse (via blood or semen): Risk factors include anal (highest risk), oral or
    vaginal sex with a partner who is a male homosexual who uses IV drugs or engages in
    anal sex, or has many sexual partners.
2. Sharing IV drug needles and syringes.
3. Babies may acquire the virus transplacentally before or during birth from an infected
    mother.
4. Breast milk may be a source for babies of infected women.
5. Hemophiliacs or recipients of many blood products prior to April, 1985.

13

A Theory of Caring: Pitfalls and Promises

Sara T. Fry

During the past 12 years, the National Caring Conferences have provided excellent opportunities to learn about recent thought and up-to-date research findings about human caring. The conferences have even developed internationally demonstrating a worldwide interest in human caring. Scholarship on the phenomenon of human caring has increased dramatically during this period of time. Because of these developments, nursing as well as other disciplines are focusing their attention on the phenomenon of human caring.

Consider, for a moment, the titles of some of the papers presented at this conference. Sally Gadow has eloquently analyzed the connections between caring and knowing, and has encouraged us to embrace a new understanding of these processes within "the land of nursing." Marilyn Ray has analyzed the research methodologies appropriate to the caring phenomenon while Westorick, Larson and Dodd, and Clayton et al. have addressed the *practice* of caring within nursing experience. These and other presentations build on and enhance the importance of early works on human caring which are found in the collections edited by Madeleine Leininger (1981a, 1984) and recently reprinted by Wayne State University Press in 1988.

Given all of these developments, it is not surprising to anyone that a theory of human caring is of renewed interest. Caring has been analyzed anthropologically (Aamodt, 1978; Leininger, 1981b), historically (Gustafson,

161

1984, Leininger, 1981d), and philosophically (Fry, 1990; Gaut, 1981, 1984; Griffin, 1983; Ray, 1981). Additionally, it has been characterized as a phenomenon (Boyle, 1984; Leininger, 1981a), a life force (Bevis, 1981), a potential science (Parse, 1981; Watson, 1981, 1985), a process (Guthrie, 1981; Uhl, 1981), a behavior (Leininger, 1984b), an ideal (Watson, 1985), a value (Fry, 1989a, b), a principle (Frankena, 1983), a virtue (Brody, 1988; Knowlden, 1990), and even the central unifying domain for the body of knowledge and practices in nursing (Leininger, 1981c, 1984b).

Given all of these acknowledged dimensions to the phenomenon of caring, can any theory of caring hope to adequately address all of these dimensions? Probably not. It is possible, however, that multiple theories of caring will emerge over the next few years. It is also possible that a pluralistic theory of caring will emerge once theorizing about caring gains momentum. The directions these theories of caring may take or the approaches to theorizing that might be utilized cannot be envisioned, at least, currently. Present work only promises that the future is very bright for nursing theorizing, in general, and certainly unlimited for theories of human caring, in particular. There are, however, a few obstacles to overcome before the promise of a comprehensive theory of caring is realized.

This paper will address the promises and potential pitfalls associated with constructing any theory of caring. First, I will review some of the traditional models of care and caring that have already appeared in the literature. Second I will explore hypothetical models of caring for the practice of nursing. Last, I will describe some of the problems that must be overcome for the development of theory that will address the many conceptual, epistemological, and moral dimensions of caring.

TRADITIONAL MODELS OF CARING

There are several ways that models of caring can be characterized. In 1990, however, I chose to characterize them as three: the cultural model, the feminist model, and the humanistic model.

Cultural Model of Caring

The cultural model, which to date appears the strongest model of caring, developed from anthropological and sociological studies of caring behaviors in various world cultures. This model, which is evident in the work of Madeleine Leininger and others, tends to relate caring to cultural beliefs, practices, and the survival of all humans. As Leininger (1984a) claims:

> The anthropologic record of the long survival of humans makes us pause to consider the role of care in the evolution of humankind. Different ecologic, cultural, social, and political contexts have influenced human health care and the survival of the human race. One can speculate that cultures could have destroyed themselves had not humanistic care acts helped to reduce intercultural stresses and conflicts and protect humans. (p. 5)

Research efforts within this model have generally attempted to uncover the caring phenomenon in cultural practices and to understand how caring is related to human health (Boyle, 1984; Dugan, 1984; Leininger, 1984b). Where such studies have included nursing or have been conducted by nurses, caring has been regarded as a phenomenon that tends to supply nursing with its uniqueness and central purpose. The science of nursing practice has even been called the science of caring (Watson, 1981).

Feminist Model of Caring

Because of the works of Carol Gilligan (1977, 1982), Nel Noddings (1984), and Kittay and Meyers (1987), the feminist model of caring has recently enjoyed much notoriety. Based, in part, on developments in ethics education, feminist theory, and social psychology, this model describes caring within a feminist perspective of moral development and cultural practices. Human caring is a phenomenon and an attitude that expresses our earliest memories of being cared for (Noddings, 1984). As a behavior, it can also be learned and nurtured in the educational process.

Those who work from a feminist perspective on caring tend to advocate a comprehensive picture of caring related to ethical behaviors and choices. Noddings (1984), for example, states that ". . . to care may mean to be charged with the protection, welfare, or maintenance of something or someone" (p. 9). For her, one cares through the modalities of receptivity, relatedness, and responsiveness.

The feminist model is very attractive to those interested in the practice of human care in nursing. It is already an implicit component of Watson's views of human caring (1985) and seems to be influencing current discussions of the caring phenomenon in many subtle ways.

Humanistic Model of Caring

This model of caring has been developed through the works of Marilyn Ray (1981, 1987), Delores Gaut (1981, 1984), Jean Watson (1985), Sally Gadow (1980, 1985) and Sr. Simone Roach (1989). These authors characterize caring as a will, a commitment, an intention, as well as an ideal. Caring is not specifically gender related, as in the feminist model, nor is it culturally related as in the cultural model. Caring is simply a mode of being that calls for a philosophy of moral commitment toward protecting human dignity and preserving humanity.

Characterizing caring as a moral obligation or duty is a second way that this model has been developed. As such, caring is an action created by the moral dimensions of a specific role toward some person(s). This view of caring can be seen in the work of physician and humanist, Edmund Pellegrino (1985), who believes that an individual has the obligation to promote the good of someone with whom he or she has a special relationship. For Pellegrino, this is precisely the type of caring that physicians and nurses are called on and expected to provide. It is a caring created by the obligation to provide good—an obligation inherent to the special relationships among health care workers and their patients.

The moral point-of-view (MPV), which is found in the works of philosopher William Frankena (1983), comprises the third model of humanistic caring. The moral point-of-view leads to theorizing about moral judgments and principles, about the differences among them, and about the general nature of their justifications (Fry, 1989a, 1989b, 1990).

To take a MPV about care means to take a view about caring or to adopt caring as the central principle of one's moral system of thought. It means, for Frankena (1983), to be non-indifferent to what goes on in the lives of people, to adopt a respect for persons, or to take an attitude of Christian love toward others. Such caring can take forms other than these but the person who cares from a MPV *subscribes* to a view of caring and then lives that view in his or her life. Living as care, of course, goes beyond merely accepting a morality of care as a guide for one's moral life.

In summary, these are the three traditional models of care and caring that have influenced contemporary discussions of the caring phenomenon. They are not inclusive and other models of care and caring undoubtedly exist and have their influences, as well. They are, however, the most prominent models that have influenced the discussion of care and caring in relation to nursing practice.

MORAL FOUNDATIONS FOR A PLURALISTIC MODEL OF CARING

In recent months, I have reconceptualized my characterizations of these traditional models in light of the increasing scholarship on caring in the nursing literature (Fry, 1989a, 1989b). Instead of a cultural, feminist, or humanistic model of caring, I now believe it more important to view our models of care/caring as inherently *obligation-oriented* or as inherently *covenant-oriented*.

There are several advantages to reconceptualizing care and caring in either of these ways. First, models of care would not be confined to particular schools of thought and narrow disciplinary aims. Instead of separating feminist from cultural and philosophical views, one could focus on the moral dimensions of caring rather than anthropological, sociological, psychological, or philosophical perspectives about caring. Second, our three models of caring would be reduced to two models that are broader in scope and that focus on the moral foundations for care and caring.

Third, obligation- and covenant-oriented models of care recognize that care and caring are always understood and practiced within some context. As Benner and Wrubel (1989) point out, caring is a form of involvement with others that creates possibilities of concern for one's world. This means that "caring (about someone or something) places a person in a situation in such a way that certain aspects show up as relevant" (Benner & Wrubel, 1989, p. 4). Some of these aspects are duties or obligations between individuals in special relationship to one another.

An *obligation* model of care highlights aspects of compassion, doing good for others, and medical competence which are all directed toward the good of an individual (Figure 13-1). One cares in order to produce some good or to create some benefit for another individual. However, I am not at all certain that nursing should adopt this model of caring even though it appears to fit the realities of the nurse–patient relationship. In fact, any theory of care developed from this model would pose the very serious problem of relegating care to an interpretation of human good. I have argued elsewhere that nurse caring does not necessarily hinge on an interpretation of human good and often, in fact, occurs where the good of the patient has not yet been determined (Fry, 1989a, 1989b).

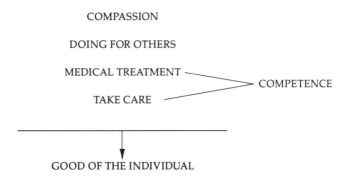

Figure 13-1
Obligation Model of Caring

It also seems that the kind of caring that nurses are familiar with tends to involve more than what is contained in an obligation model of care. Authentic nurse caring is based *not* on patient good, therefore, but on the maintenance of fidelity in the relationship with the patient. Hence, it is a *covenant* model of care.

A focus on covenant suggests that, rather than human good as the basis for human caring, fidelity is the basis for nurse caring. Fidelity between persons stems from the covenant made between persons when they stand in particular relationships to one another (Cooper, 1988; May, 1983). It includes the elements of compassion and doing for others that are contained in the obligation-oriented model (Figure 13-2). However, it also includes respect for persons and the protection of human dignity which are elements foundational to the nurse–patient relationship (American Nurses' Association, 1985).

Does this mean that competence is not related to human caring within health care relationships, especially the nurse–patient relationship? The model seems to suggest this. However, I am advised that caring and competence are closely related in the nurse–patient relationship. Indeed, empirical studies on nurse caring demonstrate that competence is an important component in the patient's perspective about how he or she is being cared for (Valentine, 1990). Perhaps the elements of competence should not be omitted from any model of caring for health care relationships. Respect for persons and human dignity, elements essential to a covenant model of care, may even lose their moral force if they are not directed with competence to the one who requires care on the part of the nurse.

COMPASSION

DOING FOR OTHERS

RESPECT FOR PERSONS

PROTECTION OF HUMAN DIGNITY

FIDELITY

**Figure 13-2
Covenant Model of Caring**

Each of these models—the *obligation* model of care and the *covenant* model of care—have a moral appeal that is legitimate if somewhat limited due to the type of relationship within which care or caring occurs. There is even reason to believe that any comprehensive approach to theorizing about care/caring may require more than a single orientation, such as obligation or covenant. Baruch Brody (1988), for example, suggests that pluralistic moral theory is desired for health care relationships and that various moral appeals can and should be components for this type of theory. This is an interesting idea and it may be beneficial to the formation of a model of caring.

A *pluralistic model of caring* might include both obligation and covenant formation. Indeed, the parties to a covenantal relationship are, in certain respects, under an obligation to behave in certain ways within the relationship. Obligation between parties, however, is not solely for the purpose of producing good. Obligation exists to define compassion between the parties of the relationship and the acts of caring that will be involved. Independence in the relationship is maintained by the other elements of the covenantal model—the elements of respect for persons and the protection of human dignity. Hence, a pluralistic model of caring contains obligation elements as well as independence elements. All elements, however, are focused on fidelity as the context within which caring becomes the possibility of giving help and receiving help.

Theory based on this type of model would necessarily identify links between several conceptual aspects of caring. Caring as a mode of being in the world insofar as caring is a natural state of human existence comprises a primary aspect here; for it is the way humans relate to their world and to each other. We find such a view of caring in the work of Nel Noddings (1984) who considers caring as a natural sentiment of being human. Noddings also calls caring a feeling or an internal sense universal for the whole species. This is the type of caring that one commonly sees between a mother and child, human or animal.

A second aspect of caring is its status as a precondition (or an antecedent) of caring about specifics. This is eloquently discussed by Griffin (1983) when she states that a conceptual idea about caring exists as a structural feature of human growth and development prior to the commencement of the caring process.

A third aspect of caring identifies it with moral or social ideals such as the human need to be protected from the elements or the need for love (Griffin, 1983). Nursing practice is linked to these moral and social ideals because caring occurs within the context of health care which serves the needs of the community. Caring, therefore, is a moral phenomenon and not simply a human phenomenon.

Given these rough characterizations of the conceptual linkages in a pluralistic model of caring and the promise of a comprehensive theory of caring in the future, several cautions and questions seem pertinent.

AVOIDING THEORY DEVELOPMENT PITFALLS

Obviously, several pitfalls must be avoided in the development of any theory of care/caring. First, there is no clear conceptual understanding of the phenomenon of human care and its various dimensions despite all of the efforts I have just reviewed and described. For example, some consider care to be a mode of moral judgment and call it either feminine or masculine. These gender-related terms are understood to connote a specific type of approach to moral decision making and the justifications for moral judgments. Many women and nurses, in particular, have focused on this interpretation of care and caring because it seems to create an enhanced sense of moral agency by touching on that which is inherently feminine. The result is a dichotomy between "the masculine voice of justice" and "the feminine voice of caring"—a dichotomy that may, in fact, be false. Accepting this dichotomy makes it difficult to determine if care and caring are important to nursing because they are related to what nurses do in patient care or because they are feminine, with most nurses obviously of the female gender. This pitfall must be avoided.

A second potential problem concerns the status of care or caring as a duty/obligation, a value, or a principle. When care/caring is associated with *duty or obligation*, care/caring is characterized as a component of the professional duty to provide good or to promote the welfare and well being of the patient. The expressed nature of the obligation between professional and patient may, in turn, be linked to several interpretations of patient good. For Pellegrino (1985), these senses of good include: (1) medical craftsmanship or what treatment can be offered to alter the illness process (p. 21), (2) whatever good the patient considers is worthwhile or in his or her best interests (p. 21), and (3) the good "most proper to being human" or whatever fulfills one's potential and expresses one's human dignity and freedom (p. 22). Caring, as a duty, is presumed to enhance these senses of patient good. Is this the type of caring that we have in mind when we speak of a theory of caring for nursing practice?

If caring is a *value*, as I have argued elsewhere (Fry, 1989a, 1989b), several aspects of caring are emphasized. The nonmoral aspects of caring become related to the activity of providing care and the attitudes or feelings that underlie the activity of providing care. The moral aspects are therefore related to the perception of need for care as expressed by the patient and the professional duty to respond to the need as recognized by the professional. As a value, caring is a human action or character trait that is deserved and preferred, and that might be formalized as *duty*, when the welfare of other humans are of concern.

If caring is a *principle*, as Frankena (1983) has argued, then caring is an action guide for our normative judgments involving other persons. Caring therefore stems from or is generated by our general attitudes toward personhood and human dignity. Expressed as a principle, caring is non-indifference about what happens to persons and is adequately expressed in Christian love or as a Kantian form of respect-for-persons (Frankena, 1983). Such caring is then justified just like any other normative judgment made by individuals. The principle of non-indifference is, for Frankena, a *lived* principle for a system of morality that can encompass all human actions.

The final problem that should be avoided in developing a theory of caring concerns defining care/caring too narrowly. In other words, is there more to care/caring than merely its status as a duty, value, or principle? Is care relational, as Sally Gadow (1985) described it? Is it an "existential phenomenon" that typically coincides with a duty to care? And if this is the case, what is the status of care/caring with regard to other moral phenomena in human practices? Deciding on any one of these interpretations of care/caring will thrust the would-be theorist into sticky philosophical debates that are often waged over these conceptual issues.

Moving into these debates is, after all, the task before us. Perhaps the papers given at this conference and the discussions thereby provoked will provide the opportunity for some persons to develop their ideas further and to actually propose a theory of care and caring in the near future. I look forward to that day.

REFERENCES

Aamodt, A. M. (1978). The care component in a health and healing system. In E. Bauwens (Ed.), *Anthropology and health*, pp. 37–45. St. Louis: C. V. Mosby Company.

American Nurses' Association (1985). *Code for nurses with interpretive statements.* Kansas City: The Author.

Benner, P., & Wrubel, J. (1989). *The primacy of caring: Stress and coping in health and illness.* Menlo Park, CA: Addison-Wesley Publishing Company.

Bevis, E. O. (1981). Caring: A life force. In M. M. Leininger (Ed.), *Caring: An essential human need*, pp. 49–59. Detroit: Wayne State University Press.

Boyle, J. (1984). Indigenous caring practices in a Guatemalan colony. In M. M. Leininger (Ed.), *Care: The essence of nursing and health*, pp. 123–132. Detroit: Wayne State University Press.

Brody, B. (1988). *Life and death decision making.* New York: Oxford University Press.

Brody, J. (1988). Virtue ethics, caring, and nursing. *Scholarly Inquiry for Nursing Practice, 2*(2), 90–97.

Cooper, C. C. (1988). Covenantal relationships: Grounding for the nursing ethic. *Advances in Nursing Science, 9*(3), 34–43.

Dugan, A. B. (1984). Compadrazgo: A caring phenomenon among urban Latinos and its relationship to health. In M. M. Leininger (Ed.), *Care: The essence of nursing and health*, pp. 183–194. Detroit: Wayne State University Press.

Frankena, W. K. (1983). Moral-point-of-view theories. In N. E. Bowie (Ed.), *Ethical theory in the last quarter of the twentieth century*, pp. 39–79. Indianapolis: Hackett Publishing.

Fry, S. T. (1989a). The role of caring in a theory of nursing ethics. *Hypatia: A Journal of Feminist Philosophy, 4*(2), 88–103.

Fry, S. T. (1989b). Toward a theory of nursing ethics. *Advances in Nursing Science, 11*(4), 9–22.

Fry, S. T. (1990). The philosophical foundations of caring. In M. M. Leininger (Ed.), *Ethical and moral dimensions of care*, pp. 13–24. Detroit: Wayne State University Press.

Gadow, S. A. (1980). Existential advocacy: Philosophical foundation of nursing. In S. Spicker & S. Gadow (Eds.), *Nursing images and ideals: Opening dialogue with the humanities*, pp. 79–101. New York: Springer Publishing.

Gadow, S. A. (1985). Nurse and patient: The caring relationship. In A. H. Bishop and J. R. Scudder (Eds.), *Caring, curing, coping: Nurse, physician, patient relationships*, pp. 31–43. Birmingham: University of Alabama.

Gaut, D. A. (1981). Conceptual analysis of caring: Research method. In M. M. Leininger (Ed.), *Caring: An essential human need*, pp. 17-24. Detroit: Wayne State University Press.

Gaut, D. A. (1984). A philosophic orientation to caring research. In M. M. Leininger (Ed.), *Care: The essence of nursing and health*, pp. 17-25. Detroit: Wayne State University Press.

Gilligan, C. (1977). In a different voice: Women's conceptions of self and of morality. *Harvard Educational Review*, 47, 481-517.

Gilligan, C. (1982). *In a different voice: Psychological theory and women's development.* Cambridge: Harvard University Press.

Griffin, A. P. (1983). A philosophical analysis of caring in nursing. *Journal of Advanced Nursing*, 8, 289-295.

Gustafson, W. (1984). Motivational and historical aspects of care and nursing. In M. M. Leininger (Ed.), *Care: The essence of nursing and health*, pp. 61-73. Detroit: Wayne State University Press.

Guthrie, B. (1981). The interrelatedness of the caring patterns in black children and caring process within black families. In M. M. Leininger (Ed.), *Caring: An essential human need*, pp. 103-107. Detroit: Wayne State University Press.

Kittay, E. F. & Meyers, D. T. (1987). *Women and moral theory.* Totowa, NJ: Rowman & Littlefield.

Knowlden, F. (1990). The virtue of caring in nursing. In M. M. Leininger (Ed.), *Ethical and moral dimensions of care*, pp. 89-94. Detroit: Wayne State University Press.

Leininger, M. M. (1981a). *Caring: An essential human need.* Proceedings of the Three National Caring Conferences. Detroit: Wayne State University Press.

Leininger, M. M. (1981b). Cross-cultural hypothetical functions of caring and nursing care. In *Caring: An essential human need*, pp. 95-102. Detroit: Wayne State University Press.

Leininger, M. (1981c). The phenomenon of caring: Importance, research, questions, and theoretical considerations. In *Caring: An essential human need*, pp. 3-15. Detroit: Wayne State University Press.

Leininger, M. M. (1981d). Some philosophical, historical, and taxonomic aspects of nursing and caring in American culture. In *Caring: An essential human need*, pp. 133-144. Detroit: Wayne State University Press.

Leininger, M. M. (1984a). *Care: The essence of nursing and health.* Detroit: Wayne State University Press.

Leininger, M. (1984b). Care: The essence of nursing and health. In *Care: the essence of nursing and health*, pp. 3-15. Detroit: Wayne State University Press.

May, W. F. (1983). *The physician's covenant.* Philadelphia: The Westminster Press.

Noddings, N. (1984). *Caring: A feminine approach to ethics and moral education.* Berkeley: University of California Press.

Parse, R. R. (1981). Caring from a human science perspective. In *Caring: An essential human need*, edited by M. M. Leininger, pp. 129-132.

Pellegrino, E. (1985). The caring ethic: The relation of physician to patient. In A. H. Bishop & J. R. Scudder (Eds.), *Caring, curing, coping: Nurse, physician, patient relationships*, pp. 8-30. Birmingham: University of Alabama Press.

Ray, M. A. (1981). A philosophical analysis of caring within nursing. In *Caring: An essential human need*, pp. 25–36. Detroit: Wayne State University Press.

Ray, M. A. (1984). The development of a classification system of institutional caring. In *Care: The essence of nursing and health*, pp. 95–112. Detroit: Wayne State University Press.

Ray, M. A. (1987). Technological caring: A new model in critical care. *Dimensions in Critical Care Nursing*, 6(3), 166–173.

Roach, Sr. M. Simone (1989). *The human act of caring: A blueprint for the health professions*. Ottawa, Ontario: Canadian Hospital Association.

Uhl, J. (1981). Caring as the focus of a multidisciplinary health center for the elderly. In *Caring: An essential human need*, pp. 115–125. Detroit: Wayne State University Press.

Valentine, K. (1990). *Nurse–patient caring: Challenging our conventional wisdom*. Paper presented at the 1990 National Caring Conference, Houston, Texas.

Watson, J. (1981). Some issues related to a science of caring for nursing practice. In *Caring: An essential human need*, pp. 61–67. Detroit: Wayne State University Press.

Watson, J. (1985). *Nursing: Human science and human care: A theory of nursing*. Norwalk, CT: Appleton-Century-Crofts.

14

Care: A Significant Paradigm Shift and Focus in Nursing for the Future

Ruth Ann Belknap

In the mid 1980s I read with interest and enthusiasm *The Aquarian Conspiracy: Personal and Social Transformation in the 1980's* (Ferguson, 1980). Ferguson describes a "leaderless but powerful network working to bring about radical change in the United States" (p. 32), which she calls the "Aquarian Conspiracy": a conspiracy for a new human agenda to bring about social renewal. Her writing describes a cultural transformation in which the emerging health paradigm places emphasis on human values and holism. Assumptions for "The New Paradigm of Health" include an emphasis on human values and the professional's caring as a component of healing (p. 247). At the time, I was impressed with how little Ferguson's writing reflected what I observed to be occurring. Medicare prospective payment had just been introduced and it seemed the world was far more concerned with cost containment and technology than with humankind and caring. Care was not perceived as having the same status as cure. Nurses, in their effort to achieve status and recognition, tended to focus on cure, fearing an association with caring for others might be demeaning (Leininger, 1984a).

This paper will explore what I believe to be a paradigm shift occurring in nursing, and will examine, as we move into the 1990s, how the concept of

173

human care is gaining recognition as a central focus and major component in the paradigm of nursing. Nurses are beginning to value care as a scientific and humanistic phenomena. As care emerges as the focus of nursing, the nurse's ability to provide compassionate human care will predominate.

Various meanings are associated with the word *paradigm*. Ferguson (1980) discussed *paradigm* as framework for thought, a scheme for understanding and explaining reality. Although new paradigms include old paradigms as partial truth, new paradigms also involve a recontextualization of what was present all along. This ability to understand phenomena in a new context is, as Ferguson (1980) explains, the process of paradigm shift itself:

> As experienced by an individual, the paradigm shift might be compared to the discovery of the "hidden pictures" in children's magazines. You look at a sketch that appears to be a tree and a pond. Then someone asks you to look more closely — to look for something you had no reason to believe was there. Suddenly you see camouflaged objects in the scene: the branches of the tree become a pitchfork, the lines around the pond a toothbrush. Nobody can talk you into seeing the hidden pictures . . . either you see them or you don't. But once you see them they are plainly there . . . You wonder how you missed them before (p. 30).

As I began to explore Leininger's nursing theory of cultural care diversity and universality, I also experienced a paradigm shift as just described. The "hidden picture" was the concept that "care is the essence of nursing and the central, dominant, and unifying feature of nursing" (Leininger, 1988b, p. 152). Ferguson describes the discovery of a new paradigm as both exhilarating and humbling, not more knowledge but a new way of knowing. So it was for me. I was excited by what felt like incredible insight, yet humbled. Clearly "care" had been central to my understanding of nursing; why had it remained invisible and not apparent as the dominant, explicit, and central focus of nursing?

I believe the answer to this question has several elements. The first element is the invisibility and devaluation of caring in our society. Watson (1990) wrote, "women's caring work is invisible, and somehow subsumed under the important work of men (medicine) in the patriarchal healthcare system" (p. 63). MacPherson (1989) discusses the difficulty of operationalizing a caring ethic in the corporate context of health care where care is not rewarded.

The second element pertains to nursing's struggle with professionalization. According to Hall (in Aydelotte, 1990, p. 10), the professions are occupations that exercise great power and influence in the wider social structure. Within the development of the profession of nursing, the struggle for power and influence has had its effect as well. Freire's (1971) model of oppressive group behavior is helpful in explaining what has happened to nursing. According to Freire, the dominant group (medicine) establishes its norms and values as the "right" ones. Subordinate groups (nursing) internalize these norms, believing that to be like the oppressor will lead to power and control. In their attempt to become like the oppressor the subordinate group begins to lose its cultural identity. Two striking examples of nursing's identification with medicine are (1) organization of nursing specialties in a pattern resembling medical specialties and (2) the willingness of nurses to take on medical tasks "that are no longer profitable, prestigious, or challenging enough for the physician," under the guise of expanded practice (Lovell, 1981). This identification with medicine has prevented nursing from focusing on caring, contributing to the loss of nursing's cultural identity as a caring service.

A third element here is the explosion of technology during and after World War II which has also had a negative impact on the development of care as a highly visible organizer of nurses' work. Modern technological equipment has taken center stage as the focus of nursing education and nurses' work. According to Leininger (1988a), American nurses have become dependent on modern technology and find it difficult to function in cultures with limited technology; schools of nursing evaluate students "mainly on these technical skills and less on human care concepts and principles"; and "the teaching of care components such as surveillance, presence, empathy, comfort, touch, and compassion has decreased in education and clinical settings since 1950" (p. 22). Thus technology, not care, has been the visible organizer of nursing's work.

During the 1980s, the corporatization of health care continued and escalated. Health care became profit making, high tech, big business, with emphasis placed on cure at any cost. The importance of supporting and ministering to people in sickness and death was overlooked. Both "the glamour of cure and the war against illness and death" (Callahan, 1990, p. 111) have distracted us from care. There has been what Watson (1985) calls "a proliferation of the 'curing syndrome' and an adoption of the cure techniques" (p. 28). In order to meet technologic and bureaucratic demands, care has received less and less attention.

As we move into the 1990s, we enter a renaissance in society now taking shape. As the world has become more industrialized and our lives more intruded upon by technology, the absence of a focus on care has served to shed light on how acutely care is needed. "The most exciting breakthroughs of the twenty-first century will occur not because of technology but because of an expanding concept of what it means to be human" (Naisbitt & Aburdene, 1990). The societal trends described by Naisbitt and Aburdene indicate that time is right for a paradigm shift in nursing. Instead of detaching from care, we are now beginning to understand that nursing's strength and power exists in nursing's ability to provide expert and compassionate professional care.

Astute nurses have always understood the centrality of care in nursing. In the early 1950s, Leininger began to focus on the phenomenon of care. She soon realized that care was "inextricably linked" with culture and that care could not be separated from culture. As she developed her theory of cultural care, she envisioned the richness, value, and power of care for nursing care actions and decisions. In order to link culture to care, however, Leininger realized she needed to understand culture. Leininger became the first nurse with graduate preparation in nursing to become a doctorally prepared anthropologist (Leininger, 1988b). Her theory of cultural care diversity and universality opened the door for a paradigm shift in nursing.

In her introduction to the first National Caring Conference, Leininger (1978) provided the following rationale for the study of caring. First, "the construct of care appears critical to human growth, development, and survival" (p. 7). Caring is a human action. Leininger took the position that cultures had depended on care for survival since the beginning of humankind, and that care was the critical factor in human growth, evolution, and survival. However, the prehistorical and historical aspects of care have not been systematically studied.

Leininger defines a second reason for studying care: the explication of caregiver and care recipient. Important questions about care—Who were the early caregivers? How was care given? Have women always been the traditional caregivers? What was caregiver status in the past?—could be answered by such studies.

Leininger cites a third reason for studying care: the need to maintain the human attribute of caring as a therapeutic and healing force of health for current and future cultures. She discusses this need in relationship to the technological emphasis that tends to depersonalize humans and deemphasize care. Technology constrains and threatens the well being and health of humanity. Clearly in order to know, use, and preserve beneficial caring we need to identify and articulate caring in nursing practice.

Last, Leininger cites nursing's neglect of the systematic study of care as rationale for such study. She contends that the forms, meanings, symbols, structure, and function of care have been studied just barely. There is need for this type of research as well as research on the transcultural dimensions of care.

Nursing has a long association with the word *care*. However, we have not defined care or differentiated care given by nurses from care given by others. Leininger's cultural care theory is knowledge generating. She views theory as "sets of interrelated knowledge with meanings and experiences that describe, explain, predict, or account for some phenomenon . . . through an open, creative, and naturalistic discovery process" (1988b, p. 154). The purpose of cultural care theory is to guide nurses in discovering the epistemological sources of nursing knowledge related to care. The ultimate goal of the theory is to allow nurses to provide culturally congruent nursing care.

Leininger's work has led to the systematic study of the nature and phenomenon of caring. Included here is a sample of studies which utilize Leininger's theoretical and conceptual framework.

In "Southern Rural Black and White American Lifeways with Focus on Care and Health Phenomena," Leininger (1984b) discovered care constructs of rural Afro-Americans and Anglo-Americans in south central Alabama. The dominant ethnocare constructs were identified as concern, presence, involvement, and touch. This study indicated the importance of identifying care values of a culture from an *emic*, or insider's, perspective.

Wenger and Wenger (1988) examined the care patterns of the Old Order Amish. Care concepts identified in this study were mutual aid and interrelatedness. Because such concepts are of central importance to the Amish, they serve as patterns of care to guide nurses' decisions and actions in providing nursing care to the Amish. These care constructs need to be preserved and promoted in giving culturally congruent care to the Amish.

Gates (1988) determined caring behaviors of couples during hysterectomy. Her study categorized behaviors in the caring domains of communication, physical facilitative, and supportive behavior. Communication behavior related to sharing feelings was identified as having major importance.

Monsma (1988) identified caring and non-caring behaviors in children of battered women. These behaviors included protective caring strategies children used to protect their mothers during abusive incidents and other self-protective caring behaviors of children. Monsma's study also identified care implications for nursing practice.

Rosenbaum (1988) conducted a study to discover the general lifeways of Soviet-Jewish immigrants who have settled in the United States and Canada since the mid 1970s. An excellent case is made for the importance of the nurse's understanding the cultural life ways of Soviet Jews in order to provide therapeutic nursing care.

Gieleghem (1988) also used Leininger's theory to examine the characteristics of couvade. This study provides a broad explanation for male involvement in pregnancy and childbirth as "protective care" (p. 125).

Further support for the position that care is now becoming a central focus and major theme in the paradigm of nursing can be found in the work of Benner and Wrubel (1989) and Watson (1985, 1990). Benner and Wrubel view caring as central to their theory of stress and coping and their theory of nursing practice. In their research they use exemplars as paradigm cases to demonstrate: (1) "the primacy of caring as the producer of both stress and coping in the lived experience of health and illness," (2) "the primacy of caring as the enabling condition of nursing practice," and (3) "the ways nursing practice based in such caring can positively affect the outcome of illness" (p. 7). Benner and Wrubel describe their shift in perspective of nursing as brought about by "understanding nursing practice as the care and study of the lived experience of health, illness, and disease" (p. 8). According to Benner and Wrubel, this shift uncovers the primacy of caring in bringing about cure, echoing Leininger's (1981) position that "there can be no curing without caring" (p. 11).

Watson (1985) believes preservation of human care to be a critical issue for nursing. She views nursing as "a human science" and human care in nursing as a "humanitarian and epistemic act" which offers promise of human preservation in society (p. 29). She views caring as the moral ideal of nursing. According to Watson, nursing has an ethical and social responsibility to be the "caretaker of care and the vanguard of society's human care needs now and in the future" (p. 32).

In a more recent article, Watson (1990) makes the case for a health care revolution that will create a new perspective on caring. She plots a shift from the "destructive, interventionist era of health care to a position that recognizes that truly natural health-illness curing and healing processes must be obeyed" (p. 65). Watson also envisions this new perspective as leading to significant challenges, some of which include: (1) giving up patriarchal structures, (2) going beyond relationships where one health care professional stands above another, (3) advocating new approaches that expand caring and healing modalities, (4) refocusing research on "caring, healing, and health processes in relationship to environmental and societal costs," and (5) transforming curricula in nursing by introducing caring morality at all levels (p. 65). However, as Leininger contends and I agree, what Watson refers to as a *revolution* is really an *evolution*.

Care scholars such as Leininger, Gaut, Ray, Horn, Watson, Benner, Wrubel, and others have contributed to the steady and dynamic unfolding of the new paradigm. The moral imperative of Watson's theme takes a posture which will support the growing evolution of the new perspective on caring.

In order to secure the new paradigm for nursing we must continue and expand nursing's efforts in caring research. Because this research involves a discovery process in a holistic framework, it demands qualitative, phenomenological, and ethnographic approaches.

"Care is the essence of nursing and the central, dominant, and unifying feature of nursing" (Leininger, 1988b, p. 152). These words embody a perspective whose time has come. I believe that in the coming decade care will become the visible work of nurses and a central organizer of the nursing paradigm. Nurses will be recognized and valued for their expertise in professional human care.

REFERENCES

Aydelotte, M. K. (1990). The evolving profession: The role of the professional organization. In N. L. Chaska (Ed.), *The Nursing profession: Turning points* (pp. 9–15). St. Louis: Mosby.

Benner, P., & Wrubel, J. (1989). *The primacy of caring*. Menlo Park, CA: Addison-Wesley.

Callahan, D. (1990). The primacy of caring: Choosing health-care priorities. *Commonweal, 117*(4), 107–112.

Ferguson, M. F. (1980). *The aquarian conspiracy: Personal and social transformation in the 1980's*. Los Angeles: J. P. Tarcher Inc.

Freire, P. (1971). *Pedagogy of the oppressed*. New York: Herder & Herder.

Gates, M. (1988). Caring behaviors experienced by couples during a hysterectomy. In M. M. Leininger (Ed.), *Care: Discovery and uses in clinical and community nursing*, (pp. 71–86). Detroit: Wayne State University Press.

Gielieghem, P. (1988). Discovery of couvade phenomenon: Theory and clinical uses. In M. M. Leininger (Ed.), *Care: Discovery and uses in clinical and community nursing*, (pp. 123–138). Detroit: Wayne State University Press.

Leininger, M. M. (1978). The phenomenon of caring: Importance, research questions, and theoretical considerations. In M. M. Leininger (Ed.), *Caring: An essential human need* (pp. 3–15). Detroit: Wayne State University Press.

Leininger, M. M. (1984a). Caring is nursing: Understanding the meaning, importance, and issues. In M. M. Leininger (Ed.), *Care: The essence of nursing and health* (pp. 83–93). Detroit: Wayne State University Press.

Leininger, M. M. (1984b). Southern rural black and white American lifeways with focus on care and health phenomena. In M. M. Leininger (Ed.), *Care: The essence of nursing and health* (pp. 133–159). Detroit: Wayne State University Press.

Leininger, M. M. (1988a). History issues and trends in the discovery and uses of care in nursing. In M. M. Leininger (Ed.), *Care: Discovery and uses in clinical and community nursing* (pp. 11–28). Detroit: Wayne State University Press.

Leininger, M. M. (1988b). Leininger's theory of nursing: Cultural care diversity and universality. *Nursing Science Quarterly, 1*(4), 152–160.

Lovell, M. C. (1981). Silent but perfect "partners": Medicine's use and abuse of women. *Advances in Nursing Science, 3*(2), 25–30, 38.

MacPherson, K. I. (1989). A new perspective on nursing and caring in a corporate context. *Advances in Nursing Science, 11*(4), 32–39.

Monsma, J. (1988). Children of battered women: Perceptions, actions, and nursing care. In M. M. Leininger (Ed.), *Care: Discovery and uses in clinical and community nursing*, (pp. 87–106). Detroit: Wayne State University Press.

Naisbitt, J., & Aburdene, P. (1990). *Megatrends 2000*. New York: William Morrow and Co., p. 16.

Rosenbaum, J. N. (1988). Mental health care needs of Soviet-Jewish immigrants. In M. M. Leininger (Ed.), *Care: Discovery and uses in clinical and community nursing*, (pp. 107–122). Detroit: Wayne State University Press.

Watson, J. (1985). *Nursing: Human science and human care*. Norwalk, CT: Appleton Century Crofts.

Watson, J. (1990). The moral failure of patriarchy. *Nursing Outlook, 38*(2), 62–66.

Wenger, A. F., & Wenger, M. (1988). Community and family care patterns of old order Amish. In M. M. Leininger (Ed.), *Care: Discovery and uses in clinical and community nursing*, (pp. 39–54). Detroit: Wayne State University Press.

15

Caring Inquiry: The Esthetic Process in the Way of Compassion

Marilyn A. Ray

INTRODUCTION

Years ago, an elderly woman bedridden with a stroke looked at me with her stark piercing blue eyes. Though I usually didn't like loud music, I turned up the radio to drown the sorrows of the sick-room I was in —to drown out the sounds and, in some strange way, the sight of the suffering one before me. Unspeaking, I looked at her. She spoke with her heart. Uncomfortable in her presence, but responding to the life of compassion deep within my heart and soul, I turned off the radio. The journey of sharing the pain that is nursing began.

I wrote this article to share ideas and an approach to method that may capture the complexity of researching caring. I have spent much time research-ing and reflecting on the nature of caring and feel intensely that it is the way of compassion, a journey of love. Caring and love are synonymous (Ray, 1981). Inquiring about caring touches the heart and translates through the soul the "speaking together" between the one caring and the one cared for. It is an immersion into the human encounter that also reveals the human, environmental, and spiritual contexts that are nursing.

The metaphorical heart and soul are the symbols and synonyms for life, living, sensitivity, reason, and integrity. These symbols represent a creative process: The gradual or, more often, abrupt shifting of consciousness from a focus on the "they" or "I" to a compassionate "we" (Kidd, 1990), which is also spiritual (that which deepens and moves one forward and upward) (Kandinsky, 1977). Compassion is a wounding of the heart by the other where the "other" enters into us and makes us other. In the minutes of presence and dialogue with the other, we have the transformative powers of the esthetic—the understanding of forms of meaning within the sheer presence of the other and of dialogue or language that exercises the most penetrative authority over consciousness (Steiner, 1989).

In the compassionate way of being, the forms of "other" in consciousness communicate a depth of felt-realness or authenticity which is intuitive (Steiner, 1989) and depends on the granting to the other to whom one communicates a share in one's being (Buber, 1965). The esthetic act in a compassionate way of being thus communicates in the understanding of forms of meaning a simultaneous immanence and transcendence—human choice to share in the life of the other, and an intuitive knowing which, as we become "other," can be translated into a call to a deeper life, a more integrated wholeness, and a coming to understand more fully what we have understood.

What does this mean for nursing and nursing inquiry? For nursing, real presence and dialogue as choice and intuition in compassionate forms of meaning in understanding is an act of creation. This esthetic act, this conceiving and bringing into being, is a birthing and growth of the divine or spiritual life within. Steiner (1989) intimated that in an esthetic act, there can be no experience which does not wager on a presence of sense that is, finally, theological. He states, "So far as it [the esthetic act] wagers on meaning, an account of the act of reading in the fullest sense, of the act of the reception and internalization of significant forms within us, is a metaphysical and, in the last analysis, a theological one"; "[t]he meaning of meaning is a transcendent postulate" (1989, pp. 215–216). Transcendence in the felt-realness of the compassionate encounter is the unwritten theology. The meaning of meaning or transcendence as unwritten theology is an apprehension of the "radically inexplicable presence, facticity and perceptible substantiality of the created, it is; we are" (p. 201) because there is creation.

For nursing inquiry as the way of compassion, the esthetic (creative) act of *knowing about* the meaning of the meaning of nursing as caring, presumes creation—the conceiving of and bringing into being a knowledge of the substantiality of the created. There is transcendence which is also theological.

There is a presence that, as the researcher dwells with the data to read "being anew" or to apprehend the nature of caring, "is the source of powers, of significations in the text, in the work [that is] neither consciously willed nor consciously understood . . . the unmastered 'thereness' of a secret-sharer, of a prior creation with and against which the art [esthetic] act has been effected" (Steiner, 1989, pp. 211–212). In essence, the felt-realness of compassion (caring) in nursing and nursing research, because of the focus on the compassionate "we," is a theological enterprise. As Emily Dickinson notes in one of her poems (Stone, 1990), "The soul selects her own society—Then, shuts the door—" (p. 9).

CARING INQUIRY: THE PHENOMENOLOGY OF ESTHETIC RESEARCH

Caring inquiry as an esthetic process in research is a unique method of presence and dialogue. It attends to both immanence—communion with and transcendence—and reflective intuition. When a researcher engages in caring inquiry, the compassionate "we" is enacted. Encountering the "other" to learn anew the world of caring and not the world as previously encoded by scientific analysis is where the word and compassion (love) interact (Steiner, 1989). Both description (phenomenology) and interpretation (phenomenological hermeneutics) and esthetic knowing of the experience of caring are the means by which questions about the meaning of caring are illuminated. Phenomenology and phenomenological hermeneutics (Van Manen, 1990) are human sciences that study persons who are experiencing the life-world. Esthetic knowing in caring research attends to creativity, sensitivity, and the quality of presences. It is an approach of describing and understanding the meaning of being and becoming through caring. In bringing to reflective awareness the nature of caring in the events experienced in the world of nursing, the researcher (and possibly the research participant) is transformed, contributing to the fullness of being and the call to a deeper life—a life of integrated wholeness and openness to creative forces within and without.

Thus, what makes phenomenological hermeneutics an esthetic enterprise is an investment of one's own being in the process of the events of the research. The response to the descriptions and interpretations of the events of caring in esthetic inquiry is one of pure receptivity and responding responsibly, or being answerable to the text in the specific sense, which is at once moral, spiritual, and psychological (Steiner, 1989). The translation of data communicated as text from "shared remembrances" of participants of the meaning of caring into the general perspective of human recognition is teaching the way of the compassionate heart and soul. It illuminates a valuation of the theological or spiritual. The phenomenology of esthetic research of caring presupposes and validates an enmeshment in the metaphysical and theological. What the method is seeking is integrity—a coming to understand more fully what we have understood—where the word and love are a synthesis.

The following is a methodological process I developed based on the ideas of Husserl, (Natanson, 1973), Van Manen (1990), Reeder (1984, 1988), and other philosophers of human science, art, and theology. The process is outlined as follows (Ray, work in progress):

1. The Intentionality of Inner Being of the Researcher.
2. The Process of Dialogic Experiencing.
3. The Process of Phenomenological-Hermeneutical Reflecting and Transforming.
4. The Movement of Phenomenological-Hermeneutical Theorizing to a Theory of Meaning.
5. Dialoguing with Written Texts: Examining Similarities and Differences.
6. Credibility and Significance of the Process of the Phenomenology of the Esthetic Act.

The general research question relates to the meaning of the experience of caring or compassion in nursing research. A specific question could be: "What is the meaning of caring in your experience?" This methodology also could be used for any other phenomenological-hermeneutical question in nursing.

THE ESTHETIC PROCESS IN CARING INQUIRY

A dynamic, disciplined, dialectical, reflective, and creative approach among the following activities forms the process of the esthetic phenomenological-hermeneutical inquiry and is outlined as follows: (Ray, work in progress)

A. The Intentionality of Inner Being of the Researcher.
   1. Imagining the vision of the caring in nursing—past and future within the present.
   2. Listening to the "voices" within embodied consciousness, as a feeling and a form of discourse about the meaning of caring in nursing.

    3. Focusing on and identifying one's presuppositions of caring in nursing.

    4. Practicing bracketing to hold in abeyance one's prehistory and presuppositions about the caring in nursing.

B. The Process of Dialogic Experiencing.

    1. Selecting the participants for the study grounded within the imagined vision.

    2. Engaging with the participants to discuss the roles of interviewer and interviewee, and securing informed consent signatures.

    3. Copresencing/sensing the other by recognizing the immediate impact of each other's being on each other—the compassionate "we."

    4. Conversing with participants in tape-recorded, intensive dialogical interviews lasting approximately one hour, about the meaning of caring in nursing by asking the phenomenological question, "What is the meaning of caring in your experience?"

    5. Engaging in a cue-taking, talk-turning, researcher-bracketed, dialogical-dialectical interactive process based on the participants' experience to penetrate the meaning of and experience how caring nursing is constructed for or understood by the other. The researcher at this time of dialogic interviewing holds in abeyance, or temporarily sets aside, his or her knowledge of caring that is a part of his or her embodied consciousness. There is continued controversy over the issue of bracketing in phenomenological philosophy (Stapleton, 1983). For the purpose of this research approach, bracketing of presuppositions about caring is used during the interviews by moving from the lead question of the meaning of experience of caring followed by the cue-taking, talk-turning interaction of the actual dialogue itself.

C. The Process of Phenomenological-Hermeneutical Reflecting and Transforming.
The Flow of Analysis occurs through:

    1. Reflecting and feeling the presencing of the participants' beings in one's consciousness.

    2. Transcribing the phenomenological data of the meaning of the art of nursing as texts through a computer-assisted data text and analytic system (Seidel, 1988).

    3. Bracketed reflecting for a pure descriptive phenomenology or receptive knowing in consciousness while engaging in the first encounter with the transcribed data (bracketing one's interpretive tendency

in relation to one's history and presuppositions about the phenomenon).

4. Attending to the speaking of language in the texts. If a transcriber,
   other than the researcher, transcribes the data, the researcher should
   listen to the tapes at the time of encountering the texts for the first
   time.

5. Highlighting the descriptive experiences of the art of nursing in the
   texts by using a highlighter pen, or device to illuminate the participants' language of experience.

6. Interpretive reflecting (hermeneutical thinking or unbracketed reflecting) to reveal the immanent themes (linguistic dimensions)
   emerging in the data. Unbracketed reflecting is the foundation for
   phenomenological-hermeneutical interpretation. Rather than brack-
   eting one's preassumptions of caring, the history or horizon of meaning of the researcher is brought into being in the dialectic of
   consciousness and the text.

7. Moving back and forth in understanding the meaning of the textual
   data to and in consciousness (copresencing and dialoguing with the
   data in consciousness).

8. Writing and transforming the themes in the transcribed text to cocreate the metathemes which are linguistic abstractions of the themes.

9. Phenomenological Reducing or Intuiting—turning to the nature of
   the transcendental meaning of the phenomenon by intuiting or grasp-
   ing the unity of meaning as a direct, unmediated apprehension of the
   whole of the experience. This is an intersubjective universal—a transcendent experience of knowing wherein the researcher as knower
   makes a connecting leap of insight and the separateness of the phenomenon melds into a whole. The universal is reached by a "coming
   together" of the variations. Thus, variations or similarities of the experience are intuitively and authentically grasped and constituted in
   consciousness—the primordial material of sensation out of which
   arises the knowing of the meaning of experience (the possibility of the
   phenomenological genesis or beginning, that is, what has been experienced as apart comes together as insight/new awareness, but is not put
   together from the different dimensions). References to the data, or
   themes, of experiences-as-meant of the meaning of caring in nursing
   from participants' experiences undergoes transformation into the researcher's intentional life, and stands out as a component of the
   researcher's concrete essence. A new way of experiencing, thinking,

and theorizing thus is opened up for the researcher. (This experience may occur at any time in the process of reflection.) A metaphor(s) may be grasped as the unity of meaning at this time.

10. Composing linguistic transformation of data to themes, metathemes or metaphor (metatheme and metaphor may be the transcendent experience).

D. The Movement of Phenomenological-Hermeneutical Theorizing to a Theory of Meaning.

1. "Putting together" a theory of meaning which, when constituted by the descriptions, themes, metathemes, and/or metaphor(s), and transcendent unity of meaning becomes the *form* or *structure* of the phenomenological meaning of caring. The theory as form may be represented as a visual model showing all the dimensions of the experience. A theory in phenomenological philosophy and method may seem contradictory given the fundamental notion of the continuous, experiencing process of the living world. However, the idea of theory in this sense is a way of giving form to the intentional acts of the research itself—where the knower and the known are one, are integral (Reeder, 1984), and where the researcher communicates to the world the integrality of understanding the esthetic act itself. Theory in this sense aims at making explicit the universal meaning of the whole of the experience. Note the etymology of theory—theo and eros—God and love.

E. Dialoguing with Written Texts: Examining Similarities and Differences.

1. Relating the theory of meaning to literary writings in art or nursing to enhance the epistemic development of nursing theory is expressed by illustrating and illuminating similarities, and differences from the phenomenological analytic data and theory or theories previously advanced. The form or structure of the meanings, i.e., the phenomenological theory, gives rise to its value in relation to the existing theories or literary works and subsequently to the implications or recommendations for nursing education, practice, administration and research.

F. Credibility and Significance of the Process of the Phenomenology of the Esthetic Act.

1. *Recognizing, believing,* and *acknowledging* are the dynamics of credibility of the research. The phenomenological evidence of the reality-as-meant of caring is what has been lived and communicated by the participants. Reality, as expressed in experience, is not inauthentic.

Meanings convince, and the meanings of the experience alter the sensibilities of those dwelling in the phenomenological written text— the researcher and other readers. Phenomenology enlarges human awareness directly or expands the range of human perception with new ways of experiencing, rather than with new, objective, mechanistic interpretations as in traditional science. Deepening and expanding the possibilities of being—the quality of making humans more human, humane, and spiritual (the ontologic), rather than more mechanistic, is the valid experience of phenomenological esthetic inquiry.

2. *Affirming* and *confirming* the meaning of the lived experience are the dynamics of significance of the research and are expressed and understood not as agreement, conformity, or generalization, but moving toward the universal which is paradoxical. The capacity to grasp and communicate the meaning of the whole of the experience is articulated and "tested" through the reflective intuition and individuality of the researcher. The universal is deep. It is a sympathetic relationship through which the researcher is transposed into the interior lives of others. The universal is undifferentiated wholeness or caring wisdom which is ultimately both within and without—a reflective symmetry, which brings together into a unity the reflective interiority of the researcher with the possibilities and contradictions of historical-cultural horizons. The quest for meaning is a social signifier and therefore exists in the relationship between the personal-mutual, the individual-community, and the specificity-commonality of culture. The movement of phenomenological theorizing to a theory of meaning captures, through the solitude of the researcher's reflection on the meaning, the researcher's capacity to bridge participants' meaning of experience of caring and the universality of human action as esthetic. Thus, the transformations or possibilities in experiencing (the epistemologic) are open or available to all readers in the reflective symmetry or synthesis encapsulated in the theory.

CONCLUSION

This article has focused on the sharing ideas and an approach to method that reflects the complexity and creative power of caring inquiry as a way of compassion and an esthetic act. What I affirmed by expressing the interiority of compassion as presence and dialogue through metaphysical and epistemological means is that caring and caring inquiry in the final analysis is spiritual and theological. The density of theological presence in nursing research has been effectively communicated by its absence in the last few decades, possibly because of the logical positivist teachings of science, or the newer dimensions of deconstructionist philosophy. It may well be that forgetting the question of the theological, in a sense forgetting to address the mystery of the hidden, yet revealed an interiority of the heart and soul that will continue to drain from nursing its creative, authentic caring potential, and the entire sphere of the esthetic—the meaning of meaning. The crisis in nursing science and practice today demonstrates an emptiness which echoes of the loss of the theological. I have communicated the loss. It could be, however, more from silence than emptiness. This article has given voice to this silence.

REFERENCES

Buber, M. (1965). *The knowledge of man.* New York: Harper and Row.

Kandinsky, W. (1977). *Concerning the spiritual in art.* (M. T. Sadler, Trans.). New York: Dover.

Kidd, S. (1990). Birthing compassion. *Weavings: A Journal of the Christian Spiritual Life, 5*(6), 18–30.

Natanson, M. (1973). *Edmund Husserl: Philosopher of infinite tasks.* Evanston: Northwestern University Press.

Ray, M. (1981). A philosophical analysis of caring within nursing. In M. Leininger (Ed.), *Caring: An essential human need* (pp. 25–36). Thorofare, NJ: Slack.

Ray, M. (work in progress). *Caring inquiry: The dialectic of science and art.* New York: National League for Nursing.

Reeder, F. (1984). Philosophical issues in the Rogerian science of unitary human beings. *Advances in Nursing Science, 8*(1), 14–23.

Reeder, F. (1988). Hermeneutics. In B. Sarter (Ed.), *Paths to knowledge* (pp. 193–238). New York: National League for Nursing.

Seidel, J. (1988). *The ethnograph.* Littleton: Qualis Research Associates.

Stapleton, I. J. (1983). *Husserl and Heidegger: The question of the phenomenological beginning.* Albany: State University of New York Press.

Steiner, G. (1989). *Real presence.* London: Faber and Faber.

Stone, J. (1990). *In the country of hearts.* New York: Delacorte Press.

Van Manen, M. (1990). *Researching lived experience.* London, Ontario: The Althouse Press.